HANDMAID TO DIVINITY

Series for Science and Culture

HANDMAID TO DIVINITY

NATURAL PHILOSOPHY, POETRY, AND GENDER IN SEVENTEENTH-CENTURY ENGLAND

Desiree Hellegers

University of Oklahoma Press : Norman

Library of Congress Cataloging-in-Publication Data

Hellegers, Desiree, 1961–
    Handmaid to divinity : natural philosophy, poetry, and gender in
seventeenth-century England / Desiree Hellegers.
        p.   cm. — (Series for science and culture; v. 4)
    Includes bibliographical references and index.
    ISBN 978-0-8061-3183-2 (hardcover)
    ISBN 978-0-8061-9407-3 (paper)
    1. English poetry—Early modern, 1500–1700—History and criticism.
2. Nature in literature.   3. Winchilsea, Anne Kingsmill Finch,
Countess of, 1661–1720. Spleen.   4. Literature and science—
England—History—17th century.   5. Religion and literature—
History—17th century.   6. Milton, John, 1608–1674. Paradise lost.
7. Donne, John, 1572–1631. Anniversaries.   8. Philosophy of nature
in literature.   9. Sex roles in literature.   I. Title.   II. Series:
Series for science and culture; v. 4.
PR545.N3H45   2000
821'.409356—dc21   99-37761
                                                            CIP

Handmaid to Divinity: Natural Philosophy, Poetry, and Gender in Seventeenth-Century England is Volume
4 of the Series for Science and Culture.

To the memory of my father, Andre E. Hellegers, and to my mother, Charlotte L. Hellegers, who taught me the three R's: reading, writing, and resistance

Nor could incomprehensibleness deter
Me, from thus trying to emprison her . . .
                                    John Donne

CONTENTS

SERIES EDITOR'S FOREWORD

In recent years, the study of science, both within and outside of the academy, has undergone a sea change. Traditional approaches to the history and philosophy of science treated science as an insular set of procedures concerned to reveal fundamental truths or laws of the physical universe. In contrast, the postdisciplinary study of science emphasizes its cultural embeddedness, the ways in which particular laboratories, experiments, instruments, scientists, and procedures are historically and socially situated. Science is no longer a closed system that generates carefully plotted paths proceeding asymptotically towards the truth, but an open system that is everywhere penetrated by contingent and even competing accounts of what constitutes our world. These include—but are by no means limited to—the discourses of race, gender, social class, politics, theology, anthropology, sociology, and literature. In the phrase of Nobel laureate Ilya Prigogine, we have moved from a science of being to a science of becoming. This becoming is the ongoing concern of the volumes in the Series on Science and Culture. Their purpose is to open up possibilities for further inquiries rather than to close off debate.

The members of the editorial board of the series reflect our commitment to reconceiving the structures of knowledge. All are prominent in their fields, although in every case what their "field" is has been redefined, in large measure by their own work. The departmental or program affiliations of these distinguished scholars— Sander Gilman, Donna Haraway, N. Katherine Hayles, Bruno Latour,

Richard Lewontin, Michael Morrison, Mark Poster, G. S. Rousseau, and Donald Worster—seem to tell us less about what they do than where, institutionally, they have been. Taken together as a set of strategies for rethinking the relationships between science and culture, their work exemplifies the kind of careful, self-critical scrutiny within fields such as medicine, biology, anthropology, history, physics, and literary criticism that leads us to a recognition of the limits of what and how we have been taught to think. The postdisciplinary aspects of our board members' work stem from their professional expertise within their home disciplines and their willingness to expand their studies to other, seemingly alien fields. In differing ways, their work challenges the basic divisions within western thought between metaphysics and physics, mind and body, form and matter.

Similarly, the volumes we have published in the series reflect crucial changes in the ways we conceive of both science and culture. In an era in which the so-called Science Wars have polarized these allegedly opposing fields of study by caricaturing both camps—"science" and "culture"—as single-minded restatements of invariant beliefs, the studies in the series elevate the level of postdisciplinary discussion by indicating ways in which we can think beyond simplistic modes of attack and defense. All coherence is not gone in a postdisciplinary era, but our conceptions of what counts as coherence, inquiry, and order continue to evolve.

ROBERT MARKLEY

West Virginia University

ACKNOWLEDGMENTS

If, for Anne Finch, Proteus is an appropriate metaphor for the mutable discourses of natural philosophy and medicine in seventeenth-century England, it also serves as an apt metaphor for this manuscript, which began years ago as a master's essay, but has much older roots in the dinner table discussions of my childhood, between my father, a physician and pioneer in the field of bioethics, and my mother, a nurse and reluctant feminist. Roland Flint and the late Michael F. Foley also contributed importantly to this study by providing early models of intellectual and creative passion. For their guidance on this project in its early incarnation as a doctoral dissertation, I wish to thank William Willeford, Sarah Van den Berg, and Eric Laguardia. I owe an infinite debt of gratitude to Robert Markley, a tireless advocate and mentor, who has read endless drafts of this work since its inception and kept me from dropping out of graduate school on numerous occasions. I am grateful to the University of Washington for a year-long graduate fellowship to Pembroke College, Cambridge University, without which the archival research that went into this study would not have been possible. I am particularly grateful, moreover, to Simon Schaffer for facilitating my residency as Visiting Scholar at the Department of History and Philosophy of Science at Cambridge and for feedback on early drafts of the chapters on Donne and Milton. I am also greatly indebted to Adrian John and Alison Winters for their insights, hospitality, and warmth during my stay at Cambridge. At various points, I have benefited from comments offered by James Bono, Ken Knoespel, Julie Solomon, Ronald Schleifer, Stuart Peterfreund, Pamela Gossin, Rebecca Merrens, Gayle Greene, Laurie Finke, and David Brande. Many thanks also to the editors of *Genre* and *New Orleans Review*, where, respectively, earlier versions of the chapters on Finch and Donne first appeared I also benefited greatly from the insights of readers for the University of Oklahoma Press, including Joel Reed. I am grateful to Alice Stanton and Kimberly Wiar of the Press for their patience, good humor, and guidance. I wish to thank Darren Higgins, Helen Burgess, Michelle Kendrick, and Harrison Higgs for their creative assistance with the cover design. Over the years, my work on the manuscript has been sustained in important ways by mentors, friends, and colleagues, including Vivian Pollak, Bob Shulman, Heidi Hutner, Laurie Mercier, David Cairns, Robert Ferguson, Carol Siegel, Dick Hansis, Wendy Dasler Johnson, Tim Hunt, Stacey Levine, Jack Stewart, Elizabeth Friedberg, Carol Swenson, Paul Remley, Millie Budny, Vickie Pfeiffer, Evan Burton, Randy Winn, Betty Redegeld, and Lisa Cummings-Harrington. Finally, without the unflagging friendship, boundless patience, and encouragement of Jen Schulz, Jean Yeasting, and my sister, Cammie Hellegers, this book could never have been completed.

HANDMAID TO DIVINITY

INTRODUCTION

Science and Culture in the Seventeenth Century

Over the last several years, critics of seventeenth-century poetry—and literary critics in general—have begun to recognize the crucial implications of developments in the history and philosophy of science for understanding the relationship between the discourses of seventeenth-century poetry and natural philosophy, and more broadly, the contemporary relationship between literature and science. Until recently, literary critics viewed "science" as a coherent theory and practice that was both objective and ahistorical. They confined themselves to examining seventeenth-century poetry as it ostensibly responded to the "revolutionary" emergence of two separate and distinct disciplines and cultures: one that encompassed the rational, verifiable "truths" of science, and another that included literary, that is, affective, aesthetic responses to the discovery of these putatively transhistorical truths. Historians and philosophers of science, however, along with critics and historians working within the emerging field of literature and science, increasingly view *science* as a term that encompasses—and in itself legitimates—a variety of interpretive strategies. These strategies, they argue, exist in a continual state of flux, of conflict and competition, responding to the concerns and values of the cultures and specific institutions in which they are produced. In this study I draw upon the works of contemporary critiques of science by historians and theorists such as Bruno Latour, Steve Woolgar, Mario Biagioli, Donna Haraway, Carolyn Merchant, Joseph Rouse, Steve Shapin, and Simon Schaffer, among others, to reevaluate the importance of seventeenth-century poetry as a critical resource for reconstructing seventeenth-century responses to the ideological implications of natural philosophy, astronomy, and medicine in the period, and for understanding the relationship between epistemological issues and power relations in contemporary Western culture.[1]

Cultural critics of science implicitly and explicitly challenge the view that while scientific claims may shape representations conventionally considered "literary," the cultural traffic is, in this sense, one-way. In examining the ways in which "scientific" claims are shaped by the broader cultural and historical matrices in which they arise, cultural critics of science problematize the distinctions between literature and science and deconstruct the binary oppositions of subject and object, reason and affect, science and aesthetics. These critics hold that science is a succession of metaphors, strategies, and disseminations of power, each of which predominates by virtue of particular political, cultural, and historical circumstances. Power, Rouse argues, is not external to knowledge; it not only influences the ways in which particular knowledge claims are deployed but also informs the very definition of knowledge itself. This view of knowledge precludes the possibility of a pure empiricism by insisting that the very selection of objects for study and the range of questions brought to bear on these objects are shaped by the preexisting concerns of the practioners of science and of the institutions in which they participate.

Cultural critics of science view scientific theories as narratives about the physical world and the human body.[2] They acknowledge the constitutive nature of representation and recognize that claims about the natural world are shaped by—and are identical to—the analogies, metaphors, and models used to describe them. Scientists, in short, do not have unmediated access to the natural world; they are no more able than the rest of us to get outside representation, to transcend language. As studies by Bruno Latour, Steve Woolgar,

Steve Shapin, and Simon Schaffer have demonstrated, scientific theories are not generated spontaneously within the laboratory space but are informed by the values of the broader cultural climate, which permeates and indeed shapes even the space of the laboratory.³ These critics and historians demonstrate that scientific narratives incorporate metaphors and values circulating within the broader culture. This view suggests, moreover, that paradigm shifts may be responses to, rather than necessarily causes of, changes in the broader cultural economy of representation, as some metaphors lose and others gain explanatory power.

It is important to emphasize at the outset that to invoke the constitutive nature of metaphor is not to argue that one story is as good as another or to diminish the instrumental value of scientific explanations. Quite to the contrary. Cultural critics and historians such as Merchant, Nancy Stepan, Rouse, and, as I argue here, Donne, Milton, and Finch recognize that in natural philosophy, astronomy, and medicine, as in poetry, metaphors have material consequences. They do not simply describe but also prescribe and *proscribe* particular interventions in and relationships to the natural world, and to the bodies of men, women, and children.

In this study, then, I wish to suggest that some of the central insights that inform contemporary cultural critiques of science are already evident in seventeenth-century England. I argue that representations of natural philosophy, astronomy, and medicine in the poetry of John Donne, John Milton, and Anne Finch reflect an awareness of and resistance to the ideologies that shape and authorize the authoritative narratives about nature, the cosmos, and the body to which these poets respond. I use the term *ideology* throughout this study to refer to ideas that both constitute and justify particular modes of sociopolitical order. If the works of these poets demonstrate a critical awareness of strategies used to mystify the ideological implications of authoritative claims about nature and the body, their critiques also necessarily register their own embodied locations in seventeenth-century English culture. Their critiques are formulated from and within their own ideological commitments and, in this respect, also register conflicts within and among these various commitments.

This seems an appropriate place to make explicit some of the ideological and material concerns that have impelled and shaped my own study. In the last few years, while completing this book, I have split my time between researching and teaching seventeenth-century English literature and science and developing an undergraduate course in American literature of the nineteenth and twentieth centuries. In my work on ecological issues in American literature, I have become increasingly aware of the work of scientists such as Wilhelm C. Hueper, Rachel Carson, and Theodora Colborn, whose research has been instrumental in calling attention to the contemporary environmental health crisis.[4] I have followed with interest the rise of the environmental justice movement, which has called into question the role that race and class play in the location and dissemination of toxic waste and chemical contaminants, and the broader failure of public health agencies to address the health concerns in these communities.[5] In researching an article on Jane Smiley's *A Thousand Acres* and the health effects of pesticide use, I became progressively aware, moreover, of the intersections that have for decades linked the cancer establishment and the pharmaceutical and petrochemical industries, and of the role that these relationships have played in the failure of the cancer establishment to spearhead broad-based research into the environmental links to cancer.[6] The weight of the evidence validating such a link was clear enough in 1964 to prompt the World Health Organization to support the claims of John Higginson, a physician and research scientist from the University of Kansas Medical Center who went on to become director of the WHO's International Agency for Research on Cancer, that the majority of incidents of cancer in humans are caused by environmental factors and thus "potentially preventable."[7] While I hope that this study will provide new opportunities for reading seventeenth-century poetry in ways that will contribute to our understanding of the cultural history of seventeenth-century England, I am more immediately invested in exploring the role that seventeenth-century poetry might play in fostering a deeper understanding of the cultural roots of the environmental crisis. The poetry of Donne, Milton, and Finch can provide readers with sophisticated models for anatomizing knowledge claims, for scrutinizing the means through which these claims are legitimated, and for delineating the ideological, political, and material goals they serve.

As I have already suggested, in its current usage the term *science* is a good deal more vexed and ambiguous in its application than we commonly recognize. However reliable the data generated by community-based epidemiological studies conducted in communities such as Love Canal, New York, and Woburn, Massachusetts, such studies are slow to be recognized as "science" until they are validated within firmly entrenched institutional structures. By contrast, studies conducted or supervised by trained professionals under the auspices of government, corporation, or university are deemed "scientific" even when they fail to generate reliable data. The term *scientific*, then, is both evaluative and descriptive and implicitly demarcates the boundaries of an interpretive elite, the institutional structures in which they are trained and socialized, and the economic interests with which they are associated.

The term *science* as we currently understand it has no precise corollary in the period under consideration. For this reason, I will refrain as much as possible from using it, except as an anachronistic abbreviation to refer collectively to the three discrete but related seventeenth-century discourses—natural philosophy, astronomy, and medicine—with which this study is concerned. Natural philosophy, astronomy, and medicine are far from seamless and monolithic discourses in seventeenth-century England. Rather, these terms encompass conflicting theories and strategies for the production, verification, and transmission of knowledge claims produced within a variety of contexts—including the university, the court, the alchemist's laboratory, the back rooms of inns, the birthing chamber, and even the kitchen. A large body of research, recently augmented by John Rogers's insightful study on seventeenth-century vitalism, demonstrates the existence of a range of epistemologies and ideologies in the period.[8] My study is specifically concerned, however, with exploring the importance of poetry as a vehicle for voicing resistance to those theories and practices that provide ideological and material support for the monarchy and for a patriarchal elite.

As Mario Biagioli, Leslie Cormack, and others have demonstrated, at the beginning of the seventeenth century, in both England and continental Europe, court patronage was beginning to play an important new role in the social legitimation of constructions of natural and cosmological order. Biagioli's comprehensive study of the important role that Cosimo de Medici's patronage played in advancing the career and claims of Galileo provides an important starting point for my own examination of the role that the politics of patronage play in shaping representations of the relationship between natural philosophy and poetry in the Jacobean court. The international prominence that Cosimo de Medici afforded Galileo's *Sidereus nuncius* from its publication in 1610 was, Biagioli has argued, due in good measure to the emblematic significance that the philosopher-astronomer assigned his discovery. The Medicean stars, Galileo suggested, provided divine authorization of the power of the Medicean dynasty. Heralded throughout Europe by the Florentian ambassadors, Galileo's "discovery" augmented the power and prominence of de Medici, but the visibility that it afforded astronomy as an instrument of statecraft was even more striking. Though, as I will suggest, Galileo's strategy for advancing his cosmological claims was far from unique, in the years immediately preceding the 1612 publication of John Donne's *Anniversaries*, the

Sidereus nuncius was a particularly important harbinger of the new roles that astronomy and natural philosophy might play in the centralization and legitimation of secular political authority. In England, where the Catholic Church no longer served as the official arbiter of claims regarding the nature of celestial and thus divine order, and where king and Parliament were engaged in a bitter struggle over the scope of the king's prerogative, arguments from natural and divine order were increasingly invoked to legitimate the unlimited authority of the monarch. The principal proponent of arguments from natural law was Francis Bacon, whose goals for the reform of natural philosophy, as Julian Martin has argued, mirror his goals for the reform of natural law in expanding and defining the king's prerogative.[9] By 1610 Bacon had already been struggling for several years to convince James to confer upon him the position of court philosopher, and with it, the power to arbitrate claims concerning natural, and thus divine, order.

If literary critics have sometimes tended to mystify the relationship between theology and science, historians of science have long recognized the intimate but vexed relationship between theology and both natural philosophy and astronomy in the early modern period. Following the Reformation, the politics of scriptural interpretation became the locus of controversy as it became increasingly clear that the capacity of the individual to interpret scripture by means of the "inner light"—the claim that underwrote Protestant theology—could serve as a justification for challenging both political and theological authority.[10] Christopher Hill has suggested that "the essence of protestantism—the priesthood of all believers—was logically a doctrine of individualist anarchy."[11] Robert Markley has argued that the crucial quest of Boyle and Newton, along with other members of the Royal Society, was to circumvent the controversy over biblical interpretation by locating in nature evidence of a divine order, which could then be used to legitimate a hierarchical society.[12] I argue that this goal also underlies Bacon's plan for the

reform of natural philosophy—and of both nature and language—
and explore Bacon's articulation of these goals in *The Advancement of
Learning* (1605).

Bacon, and subsequently members of the Royal Society including
Robert Boyle and John Wilkins, continued to view the natural
world as providing confirmation of "divine truth"; like their
contemporaries, they regarded the natural world as Second Scripture.
To a greater degree than Bacon, the members of the Royal Society
viewed the Book of Nature as supplementing, and therefore sub-
ordinate to, Scripture. However, in a cultural context in which the
Bible was invoked both to authorize and subvert every aspect of
sociopolitical order, the scope of the authority that the new
philosophers claimed in interpreting this ostensibly auxiliary and
secondary text was, at least theoretically, all-encompassing. In the
seventeenth century, then, the disputes over the nature of the
physical world are both implicated in and extend the debates over
biblical interpretation and over the nature of language itself.

As recent studies by James Bono and Robert Stillman on
seventeenth-century language projection schemes have indicated,
Bacon's natural philosophy must be viewed in the context of a wider
preoccupation with recuperating an originary Adamic language that
was implicated, along with nature, in the fall of man. Though
Bacon believed that the originary Adamic language that reflected
perfect knowledge of creation has been irredeemably lost, it
nevertheless served as the model for Bacon's idealized natural
philosophy that would unambiguously disclose the true character of
things in the world as revealed through systematic experimentation
and study of the particular elements of creation. In *The Advancement
of Learning*, Bacon represents natural philosophy as the "servant" or
"handmaid" to God, and the natural philosopher as the new apostle
whose authorized readings of the Book of Nature, and whose
technological miracles, will provide an antidote to skepticism and,
implicitly, to theologically based challenges to the authority of the

king. Bacon's experimental natural philosophy would therefore render the natural philosopher the ultimate arbiter of divine truth and ideological purity.

Bacon and subsequently members of the Royal Society held, however, fundamentally equivocal views of the natural world. If nature was inscribed with divine order, it was also corrupt and chaotic, implicated along with language in the fall of man. While the former view sanctioned natural philosophy as a pious enterprise and conferred divine authority upon the order that the natural philosopher located in the Book of Nature, the latter view paradoxically cast the technological transformation of nature as an act of redemption that restored nature to its originary state of divine order.

Bacon's representations of feminized nature, as Merchant has argued, emphasize the fallenness and corruption of the natural world. His descriptions of experimental inquiry, she suggests, reverberate with images drawn from the interrogation and trial of accused witches at the beginning of the seventeenth century. For Bacon, nature was a licentious woman whose corrupt sexuality necessitated the technological reformation of the male experimentalist. In Merchant's analysis, and in subsequent accounts by Evelyn Fox Keller and more recently Mark Breitenberg, Bacon's feminized representations of nature, which permeate the writings of the Royal Society, sanction the exploitation of natural resources in both England and the New World, while reinforcing the need to maintain custodial control over women's minds and bodies.[13]

Perhaps the most influential study of the last two decades in the challenges that it poses to positivist accounts of the history of science, Steve Shapin and Simon Schaffer's groundbreaking study *Leviathan and the Air-Pump* has provided critical insights into the ideologies and material practices that shaped and defined the experimental strategies and protocols of the all-male Royal Society.[14] Boyle's experiments with the air pump have traditionally been invoked as providing the prototype of systematic experimental inquiry. Shapin and Schaffer demonstrate, however, that Boyle's strategies for the production and verification of natural knowledge—in short, for manufacturing consent—did not present themselves as transhistorically self-evident but rather were shaped and legitimated by and within the Royal Society's self-selecting community of practioners over and against competing epistemologies. Shapin and Schaffer have argued that "disciplined collective social structure of the experimental form of life" would establish and "sustain" the "conventional basis of proper knowledge."[15] The community of experimentalists who would determine what constituted "proper knowledge" was, however, limited to male members of the upper classes, who were alone deemed qualified to witness and legitimize experimental procedures and results. Then as now, the ostensibly "public space" of the laboratory was, as Shapin and Schaffer have emphasized, anything but. The epistemology and knowledge claims produced within the closed space of the laboratory marginalized and delegitimated alternative epistemologies and interpretations of nature and the competing ideologies and material interests with which they were associated.

Importantly, Shapin and Schaffer's study does not seek to distinguish the ideological and social construction of Boyle's method from that of contemporary "objective" procedures for scientific investigation. In fact, sociological studies of the contemporary laboratory environments by Latour and Woolgar explore the ways in which claims are "transformed from . . . issue[s] of hotly contested discussion" into "well-known, unremarkable and noncontentious facts."[16] Ostensibly ahistorical scientific "discoveries" are better understood, they argue, as artifacts that are shaped by the material conditions of the laboratory environment, including the codes of behavior and strategies of inquiry into which scientists are socialized during their professional training.[17]

The writings of members of the Royal Society, like those of Bacon, reflect fundamentally contradictory views of the natural world. In *The Excellency of Theology, as Compar'd with Natural Philosophy*, Boyle applies the trope of the handmaid to articulate the complex relationship between theology and natural philosophy. Nature, wrote Boyle, ought not to be seen even as "an Handmaid to Divinity, but rather as a Lady of Lower Rank."[18] The liminal position of nature as the "Handmaid to Divinity," as I argue in chapter 3, is suggestive of the struggles of Boyle and other members of the Royal Society to reconcile its conflicting projects and ideologies, in which nature is alternately identified with the will of a dematerialized and disembodied God and with a seductive and sexualized natural world whose subordinate status opens "her" to the exploitation of the natural philosopher.

The trope of the handmaid, moreover, unwittingly calls attention to the natural philosopher's claims about nature as cultural constructions that reflect and reinforce his own ideological presuppositions and material interests, and implicitly impel the technological transformation of nature. For both Bacon and Boyle, the Book of Nature is imprinted with the divinely decreed hierarchies of gender and class. Insofar as interpretations of the Book of Nature were seen as supplementing the authority of scripture in the period, they were also viewed, as my readings of poems by Donne, Milton, and Finch suggest, as participating in broader debates concerning the scope of monarchical authority, the use and distribution of natural resources, and the nature and rights of women.

One of the most striking features of both *The Masculine Birth of Time* and *The Advancement of Learning* is the vitriolic tone with which Bacon attacks rival systems of natural philosophy, including the theories of Paracelsus and William Gilbert, whose representations of the earth as a feminized lodestone or magnet earned him the position of court philosopher to Elizabeth. *The Masculine Birth of Time*, written in 1602 or 1603, may be read as eagerly anticipating the opportunity to succeed Gilbert and replace his philosophical system with a virile philosophy that would lend crucial ideological support to the male monarch who would follow Elizabeth to the throne. Bacon's apparent immunity to attacks similar to those he directs against Paracelsus and Gilbert ought not be seen as a measure of the broad acceptance that his theories earned. Though James never conferred upon him the encompassing authority Bacon envisions for the natural philosopher in *The Advancement of Learning* and, most conspicuously, in *The New Atlantis*, any attacks on Bacon's proposals for the "reform" of natural philosophy may nevertheless have been viewed as challenging the authority of the monarch. Those who live "under hard lords of ravening soldiers," as Sidney suggests in *An Apologie for Poetrie*, had best voice their resistance only "under the pretty tales of wolves and sheep."[19] Bacon viewed metaphorical ambiguity with suspicion and, as Robert Stillman has aptly noted, regarded the poet as an "epistemological criminal."[20] Bacon's suspicions were not, moreover, entirely unfounded.

It is only logical that some of the most metaphorically complex and ambiguous verse in the history of English literature should have been produced in a period in which survival for many was contingent upon mastering the art of equivocation. These poets' complex critiques of the discourses of early modern science were forged under enormous ideological pressure. A poetics that could embody multiple and conflicting meanings was the ideal discourse for registering resistance to truth claims which, as I will argue, were authorized and legitimated at least in part because of the ideo-logical and material role they might play in advancing the power of the monarch and the interests of a patriarchal elite.

There is, I believe, no poet in the English language more adept at the science of manipulating metaphor than John Donne, and the *Anniversaries* must surely number among the most ambiguous and complex poems in English literature. I have selected the poems for close consideration because they frequently have been invoked as a representative response to the New Philosophy, as heralding the moment of an ostensibly cataclysmic cultural disruption that has come to be known as the Scientific Revolution. The poems demonstrate the complex interrelationship that links the discourses of theology and natural and political philosophy in the seventeenth century. They provide an important commentary on the role that the politics of court patronage were beginning to play in legitimating models of natural order that buttressed the power of church and monarch.

In chapter 1, to introduce my reading of the poems, I examine the historical relationship between Donne and Bacon to establish the poet's awareness of the ideological implications of Bacon's natural philosophy. While in chapter 2 I explore textual parallels between the *Anniversaries* and *The Advancement of Learning* that provide strong indications that the poems are a specific response to Bacon's proposals for the reform of natural philosophy, my argument does not by any means rest upon these parallels. Rather, my primary concern is to establish the poems' strong evidence of Donne's understanding of and resistance to the ideological commitments associated with Baconian natural philosophy, that is, to the discursive and material roles that natural philosophy and astronomy threaten to play in expanding the scope of monarchical authority.

In recent years, studies by Jeanne Shami, Paul Harland, and others have suggested that the Dean of St. Paul's may have used his pulpit when possible to contest James's absolutist claims, insisting upon the sovreignty of individual conscience and the ultimate sovereignty of God over king. My principal concern in this study, however, is with the politics of the poet from roughly 1610 to 1612, the years in which the *Anniversaries* were written and reluctantly published. The poems, I argue, demonstrate Donne's profound mistrust of monarchical authority and of the authority of both cleric and natural philosopher. For the poet of the *Anniversaries*, who is unable to envision any "station" in the Jacobean court economy that might be "free from infection," the authority of the natural philosopher is closely identified with that of the "spungy slack

Diuine." Both "Drinke and Sucke in th'Instructions" of the king
and "for the word of God, vent them out again."[21]

I argue in chapter 2 that the feminine mutability that is so
prominent a feature in the poetry of the young court rake, the
libertine Donne, assumes positive implications in the *Anniversaries*.
Donne's shadowy "she" serves as an emblem of resistance to projects
for policing representation and interpretation and for transforming
the natural world into an emblem of monarchical power. Insofar as
"she" is associated with the mystery and transcendence of a God
who will not be named, "she" resists Baconian arguments for
"redeeming"—and exploiting—the ostensibly corrupt text of the
Book of Nature. The *Anniversaries* depict a world that exists in a
state of perpetual narrative revolution, in which the metaphorical is
(con)fused with the literal, the pseudo-literal deconstructed and
reconstructed as a narrative about deconstruction and reconstruc-
tion *ad infinitem*. The multiple identities "she" can be made to
embody demonstrate the futility of attempting to provide definitive
readings of the Books of Nature and Scripture and dramatize the
chaos that these coercive interpretive strategies engender.

At the same time, the poems provide a sardonic reflection on the
poet's own investment in the economy of court patronage. The
Anniversaries explore and undermine the claims of astronomer and
natural philosopher who alternately invoke and mystify the material
and political benefits of their practices to secure privileged
positions within the economy of court patronage. In the ironic
logic of the exiled and would-be phoenix, Donne's simultaneous
insistence upon the contingency of his own verse and his willing-
ness to acknowledge his own dependency on the courtly economy
of patronage are transformed into an argument for his own
privileged place at court.

While Donne's primary concern appears to lie in preserving the
freedom and privileges of a masculine elite, Milton's critique of
royalist natural philosophy is more inclusive. In chapter 3 I explore

the dialogue on astronomy in book 8 of *Paradise Lost* as it is informed by the politics of a poet who was rabidly anticlerical and narrowly avoided execution for his persistent defense of regicide. For Milton, the authority that members of the Royal Society claimed to interpret the divine order in nature was wholly incompatible with his belief in the priesthood of all believers and with the "Liberty of Conscience" that he associates with the individual's right to search for the "revealed Will" of God in Scripture. Milton's dialogue on astronomy, I argue, explores and resists the intersecting ideologies of monarchical, class, and patriarchal privilege that shape the claims and projects of the Royal Society.

I explore the dialogue as it marks in particular key areas of ideological contention between the poet and John Wilkins, vice-president of the Royal Society and one of the society's most outspoken proponents of astronomical study. Wilkins's *The Discovery of a World in the Moone, or A Discourse Tending to Prove That 'Tis Probable There May Be Another Habitable World in That Planet* (1638) and *A Discourse Concerning a New Planet* (1640), together with Alexander Ross's *The New Planet, No Planet*, as Grant McColley first argued in 1937, serve as the principal textual sources of the dialogue. I contrast the ideology that informs Wilkins's language projection scheme and his writings on both natural philosophy and astronomy to the reformist goals pursued by the Hartlib circle during the interregnum. Astronomy serves as an example of and metaphor for speculative sciences, and for studies of natural and cosmological order that undermine the republican ideals of the revolution and advance the ideological and material interests of the monarch and the leisured classes. Together with book 9, the dialogue offers a political and theological imperative for applied sciences to serve the interests of yeoman farmers and thereby ameliorate the material conditions of the English poor.

Book 8, I argue, implicitly scrutinizes, moreover, the Royal Society's exclusion of women from the production of knowledge claims about the natural world. Eve serves in books 8 and 9 as the principal spokesperson for the applied science of husbandry. As such, she is alternately identified with an ethos of environmental stewardship and reverence for the natural world and its inhabitants, and with the ethos of an emergent capitalist economy that the poet represents as both aggressive and exploitative. Insofar as Eve is herself identified with nature, the dialogue between Raphael and Adam can also be seen as probing the role that theological readings of the Book of Nature play in justifying the subjugation and exploitation of the natural world.

Milton's dialogue on astronomy and Anne Finch's "The Spleen," the focus of chapter 4, both critique important rhetorical and methodological strategies that served to legitimate the Royal Society's interpretations of nature and support their claims to ideological neutrality. By 1662 claims to epistemological certainty were increasingly associated with Cartesian mechanism and Hobbesian materialism, both of which were seen as advancing absolutist ideologies. In contrast to an experimental method in which the validation of truth claims, gleaned through an ostensibly empirical methodology, was effected through common assent, Hobbes's natural philosophy would be modeled upon a geometrical logic; "truth" was constructed and imposed—and the multiple and subversive meanings associated with metaphor outlawed—by monarchical fiat. For English voluntarists, Hobbesian and Cartesian natural philosophy both evoked the specter of absolutism and of scriptural authority displaced. To distance themselves from the totalizing claims of Hobbes and Descartes, and from their suspect ideologies, members of the Royal Society adopted a rhetoric of probability and contingency to establish the validity of their claims. As Shapin and Schaffer have observed, "the literary display of a certain sort of morality was a technique in the making of matters of fact. A man whose narratives could be credited as mirrors of reality was a modest man; his reports ought to make that modesty visible."[22] The rhetoric of experimental "modesty," of probability and contingency, then, can be seen as an instrument in the legitimation of the claims and ideologies of the Royal Society.[23] Milton's dialogue on astronomy, I argue, demonstrates the tenuousness of the line between probability and certainty, between the narrative discontinuity that ostensibly preserves interpretive freedom and the narrative closure associated with hegemony and political absolutism.

In chapter 4, I argue that Finch's "The Spleen" explores the role that the discourse of the spleen—and more broadly the misogynist rhetoric that permeates both seventeenth-century natural philosophy and medicine—played in the increasingly heated debates surrounding women's education and writing, and in justifying women's containment within the domestic sphere. Feminist criticism in the history of science has demonstrated that the consolidation of medical practitioners within an exclusively male medical establishment had far-reaching cultural effects.[24] Thomas Laqueur and Londa Schiebinger have explored the role that cultural and historical contexts played in the construction of sex in early modern Europe and in the debates surrounding the nature and status of women in the late seventeenth and eighteenth centuries. The studies of both Laqueur and Schiebinger are important, not only because they demonstrate the dangers of sexist deviations from an empiricist methodology, but because they also demonstrate that pure empiricism is itself a myth.[25] Schiebinger has demonstrated that, measured against the anatomical ideal of the male body, the female body was regarded as inherently pathological. Studies of the discourse of hysteria by Catherine Clement, Hélène Cixous, Sandra Gilbert, and Susan Gubar have, moreover, examined the role that medical discourse played in marginalizing women's writing in the nineteenth and twentieth centuries.[26] The medical discourse of the spleen, I argue in this chapter, extended the strategy, evident throughout seventeenth-century poetry, of authorizing masculine liberty and legitimating constructions of masculine reason in opposition to feminine promiscuity and irrationality.

"The Spleen" depicts the gendered terminology of late seventeenth-century nervous disorders as a protean discourse that continually revises its strategies of oppression. In this respect, the ode provides important insights into the coercive implications of the rhetoric of contingency that framed late seventeenth-century natural philosophy. Finch's representation of masculine medical discourse and natural philosophy as "Proteus," Ruth Salvaggio has noted, bears significant resemblances to Michel Serres' contemporary descriptions of scientific discourse.[27] Serres envisions scientific discourse as composed of shifting configurations or "islands" of order that are defined in opposition to the "noisy poorly understood disorder of the sea."[28] Order in scientific theories, Serres suggests, is created in opposition to, and through the suppression of, an alien and disorderly "other." As Salvaggio has pointed out, "The Spleen" dramatizes the central role that woman plays as the embodiment of the "other," the irrational, chaotic element that Western science seeks to contain and against which it defines itself.[29] I argue that Finch's ode responds to the masculinist anxiety that underlies the discourse of the spleen by transforming this discourse into an image of feminine mutability, problematizing in the process the distinction between science and poetry.

While this study focuses explicitly on poetic critiques of royalist and masculinist ideologies in these three discourses, my purpose is not to insist upon the inherently hegemonic and masculinist character of scientific theory and practice, or for that matter, to argue for the relative nature of all knowledge claims. As we increasingly confront the toxic consequences of the Baconian faith in man's capacity to secure certain knowledge of and mastery over nature, it is important to acknowledge the urgent need for faithful accounts of a "real" world, for preserving a concept of objectivity that can provide an adequate foundation for environmental accountability and for addressing the environmental crisis. At the turn of the twenty-first century, understanding the cultural and economic matrices in which scientific claims are shaped and legitimated, and the ideological and material goals that individual claims and practices advance, is an essential element of scientific literacy. And scientific literacy is an essential survival skill in an era in which corporate-sponsored scientific studies are routinely invoked to mystify the health effects of industrial contaminants in communities from Long Island to Bhopal. My hope is that the poetry of John Donne, John Milton, Anne Finch, and others may contribute to a greater understanding of "scientific" claims as "claims on people's lives,"[30] and as claims that have had—and continue to have—a very material and critical impact on the ecosystems on which we depend.

1

FRANCIS BACON AND THE ADVANCEMENT OF ABSOLUTISM

Though the *Anniversaries* have traditionally been read as marking the breakdown of the cultural and cosmological coherence of the Renaissance in the wake of the New Philosophy and as attacking the corruption of the Jacobean court and the politics of patronage, critics have consistently treated these issues as discrete and unrelated concerns and explored them only through select passages.[1] While I share Arthur Marotti's belief that the poems, written to commemorate the first and second anniversaries of the death of the nearly fifteen-year-old daughter of the poet's soon-to-be patron, Robert Drury, and his wife, Anne, the niece of Francis Bacon, reflect Donne's frustration at his decade-long struggle to secure advancement within the patronage economy of the Jacobean Court, I do not share his belief that the poet treats the New Philosophy as little more than a peripheral joke. Donne's concerns with the New Philosophy and with the politics of patronage and, more broadly, of the Jacobean court, must be understood in relationship to one another. I seek to demonstrate, through a broad and integrative reading of the *Anniversaries*, that these intersecting concerns are interwoven throughout the poems. The *Anniversaries* explore the ways in which the quest for royal patronage defined the claims, goals, and methodologies of natural philosophy and astronomy in the early seventeenth century. The poems undermine the authoritative claims to knowledge of the divine order in nature that royalists—and most visibly Francis Bacon—increasingly invoke in the first decades of the seventeenth century to legitimate their absolutist ideology.

With the publication of *The Advancement of Learning* (1605) and *The Wisedome of the Ancients* (1609), Bacon established himself as the spokesperson for an unprecedented plan to create a state-supported scientific elite whose claim to a privileged knowledge of the divine order revealed in nature could be used to justify the unlimited expansion of the king's prerogative. Any challenges to the authorized "truths" of the natural philosopher, operating under the auspices of the monarch, would be marginalized, politically neutralized as "poetic fictions." In contrast to the deceptively simple distinction that Bacon invokes between science and poetry, Donne problematizes any clear division between these two domains in the *Anniversaries*. If for Montaigne philosophy was but "sophisticated poetry," for Donne poetry is the highest form of philosophy. In contrast to a natural philosophy that denies the mediating role of metaphor and the limitations of the human interpreter, poetry provides a model for human knowledge and creation—and for good government. In the world of the *Anniversaries*, the poet, who acknowledges the contingency of his claims, who embraces and celebrates the dialogical nature of representation, the capacity of metaphor to embody multiple and conflicting interpretations, also undermines attempts to monopolize truth and power. Donne's animosity toward Bacon, with whom he shared the patronage of Thomas Ellesmere, is evident in the *Courtier's Library* and in his marginal notes to *Bacon's Apology in Certain Imputations Concerning the Late Earl of Essex*. The *Anniversaries* represent the New Philosophy as a new ideological weapon in the conflict between Parliament and James over the scope of the king's prerogative. As such, the poems provide a geneology of Western science, of knowledge claims and technological capabilities that are legitimized insofar as they justify and facilitate the hegemonic ideologies of state interests.

I

Donne's early identification with Catholic dissenters gave him good reason to have followed Bacon's political career from its early stages with interest. Through his association with the Puritan circle at Leicester House and with his patron Sir Francis Walsingham, by 1596 Bacon was awarded a warrant to torture prisoners; such warrants, as Julian Martin has noted, "were extremely rare in early modern England." The warrant indicates the trust that the queen and her counselors placed in Bacon and the extent to which, by 1596, Bacon was already "intimately associated with the security of the queen and the regime."[2]

Donne, whose brother was arrested for harboring a priest and who later died of the plague in Newgate in 1593, would have been well aware of the brutality to which suspected conspirators were subject. The execution of the priest, one William Harrington, was presided over by Topcliffe, who was the subject of one of Donne's bitterest attacks in *The Courtier's Library*, a collection of acerbic comments on his more visible contemporaries at court.[3] Prisoners suspected of plotting against the monarch were typically subjected to prolonged sleep deprivation, "disjointed on the rack," and "rolled up into balls by machinery," until, as Robert Southwell recorded, "'the bloud sprowted out at divers parts of their bodies.'"[4] John Carey notes that between 1595 and the end of Elizabeth's reign, a hundred priests and fifty lay Catholics were executed by the Crown, most of them subjected to what Carey describes as "makeshift vivisection."[5] Despite his own apostasy, it seems unlikely that Donne could have dismissed Bacon's role in the torture and execution of Catholics. Rather, the poet would have seen his eagerness to persecute Catholics as an indication of the lengths to which Bacon would go in order to advance his position at court. The crown policy that Bacon was charged with enforcing, in any case, provided Donne with ample evidence of the importance of placing limits upon the monarchical authority that Bacon sought to enlarge.

Donne's own thwarted quest for patronage and courtly preferment gave him another good reason to focus his frustrations on Bacon. Bacon had already enjoyed six years under the protection of Robert Devereux, earl of Essex, by 1597, the year Donne began his unsuccessful suit for the earl's patronage. Together with Robert Drury, Donne had served under Essex on the 1597 expedition to Cadiz. Donne's attempts to attract the attention of Essex are evident, Carey notes, in the young poet's epigram on Sir John Winfield, with its praises for "our Earle."[6] Though he failed to secure the patronage of Essex, his friendship with the younger Thomas Egerton paved the way for Donne to secure the patronage of his father, Lord Ellesmere, Keeper of the Great Seal, on the poet's return to England.

In his capacity as secretary to Egerton, Donne would have had ample opportunities for contact with Bacon during this period, as Bacon was also under the protection of Ellesmere. A brief survey of the careers of Egerton's secretaries demonstrates that the appointment likely marked Donne out as a rising star in the circles of courtly power and influence. George Carew, who went on to become ambassador to France and Master of the Court of Wards, also served early in his career as secretary to Egerton, while Egerton's chaplains, John King and John Williams, ascended to the respective positions of bishop of London, and Lord Keeper and subsequently archbishop of York.[7] Donne's career was to follow a decidedly more circuitous and troubled path as a consequence of his marriage to Anne More. The daughter of the Commons MP George More, Anne had been living under the protection of Egerton. The marriage resulted in Donne's dismissal from Egerton's services and earned the poet-courtier a short stay in the Tower of London. It also effectively marred Donne's reputation, erasing whatever prospects he might have had for royal patronage.

While Ellesmere continued to play a central role in the advance-
ment of Bacon's legal career throughout the decade, Donne was
exiled to Mitcham. From his relative retirement there, Donne tried
repeatedly to cultivate the support of various prominent patrons in
the Jacobean court, including the Countess of Bedford, but his
attempts to secure an office were unsuccessful. As Marotti and
others have argued, the *Anniversaries'* acerbic commentary on the
politics of patronage in the Jacobean court reflect in some measure
the poet's frustrated circumstances in 1611 and 1612, and perhaps his
distaste at the lengths to which he was forced to compromise
himself in his quest for preferment.[8] Donne's frustrated quest for
patronage is a motivating factor in his exploration in the *Anniversaries*
of the role that the politics of patronage play in advancing the New
Philosophy. For Donne—and possibly for Robert Drury himself—
Bacon's career may have served to demonstrate the corrupting and
divisive effect of court ambition and, in this respect, may have
compensated the poet for his own marginalized position. Bacon is
particularly targeted for criticism in *The Courtier's Library*, earning a
unique double entry for his betrayal of his former patron Essex.
One of the entries, entitled "Brazen Head of Francis Bacon:
Concerning Robert the First, King of England," combines a
reference to Roger Bacon with an allusion to Bacon's role in the
prosecution of Essex. Donne undoubtedly would have been aware
of the image of the brazen head in Robert Green's play, *Friar Bacon
and Friar Bungay*, which depicts Roger Bacon as a megalomaniacal
magus. The allusion in Donne's entry, then, provides a critique of
both Bacon's political ambitions and of the emphasis that, like the
thirteenth-century magus, Bacon placed on technology in harnes-
sing the power of nature. The title of the entry also refers to
Edward Coke's conclusion in his legal argument against Essex, in
which he charges Essex with "affect[ing] to be Robert the first of
that name King of England." The second entry, "The Lawyer's
Onion, or The Art of Lamenting in Courts of Law, by the Same,"[9]

strikes at Bacon's hypocrisy, and indeed at the hypocrisy and theatricality of the legal system in general, which Donne had witnessed firsthand at Lincoln's Inn.

While many historians have been quick to minimize Bacon's involvement in the trial of Essex, and thus to legitimize his account in his *Apology in Certain Imputations Concerning the Late Earl of Essex*, published in 1604 to deflect the criticism that his role in the trial had engendered, Jonathan Marwil notes that Bacon was hardly a reluctant participant in the prosecution: Bacon "stepped in at a critical moment and saved Coke from thoroughly muddling the Crown's position."[10] Though Donne's personal and political loyalties to Essex are unclear, it does seem evident that Bacon's participation demonstrated a level of ambition that was remarkable even within Elizabethan court culture and provided further indication of the lengths to which Bacon was willing to go to uphold the power of the monarch in order to secure himself some part of it.[11] On the title page of his copy of the *Declaration of the Practises and Treasons Committed by Robert, Late Earle of Essex* (1601), the record of the trial drafted by Bacon, Donne scrawled a reference to 2 Samuel 16:10: "Sinete eum Maledicere nam Dominus iussit," which Bald renders as "Let him curse even because the Lord hath bidden him." The allusion may serve not simply as Donne's sardonic condemnation of the hypocrisy of what Bald terms the "vehemence of Bacon's denunciation of his former patron" but also as a critique of Bacon's increasingly vocal role as a spokesman for monarchical absolutism.[12] For Bacon, Donne seems to suggest, the monarch has replaced God as ultimate authority.

Bald observes that Drury himself "was clearly of the Essex faction" and was "well aware of the unceasing struggle for power that went on at the court, and without the least hesitation attributed the basest of motives to his opponents." Drury may, moreover, have had other reasons for sharing Donne's sentiments toward Bacon. Sir Nicholas Bacon, Drury's father-in-law, the brother of Francis Bacon, held the crown lease on Drury's land from 1593/4 until 1605 and assumed considerable debts on Drury's behalf during those years. While Drury finally gained complete control over the estate at the age of thirty-one, the tension between the two evidently escalated sufficiently that at one point Sir Nicholas sought arbitration against Drury.[13] It is quite possible, then, that Drury may have had similarly strained relations with Francis Bacon even prior to the trial and execution of Essex. If Drury himself perceived Bacon's program for the reform of natural philosophy as coming under attack in the *Anniversaries*, he may, in fact, have been all the more pleased with the poems.

II

The problem of defining the relative powers of the king and Parliament reached a crisis in the period from 1603 until the Civil War. In the early seventeenth century few, whether royalists, Puritans, or other members of the opposition in Parliament, challenged the "divine origin or sanction of kingly authority"; at the same time, however, there was, as Margaret Judson notes, an overwhelming belief that "the King's authority was limited in many ways by the law, the constitution, and the consent of man." The prerogatives or domains of the king were understood to be three: the "special privileges accorded the king in the law courts," his powers as "chief feudal lord in the kingdom," and his powers as head of state. The latter two categories were the subjects of particular controversy in the early seventeenth century. The right to private property and the rarely questioned belief that taxes were a free offering by Parliament to the king coexisted uneasily with the king's status as "chief feudal lord," a status that granted him at least theoretical ownership of all the land in the kingdom and the liberty to raise revenues and levy taxes. The latter right was a perpetual source of tension between James and Parliament. The third dimension of the prerogative included calling and dismissing Parliament, coinage and control of industries, and the authority to make "appointments to the council, the law courts, other departments of government and to the church." Judson notes that the "spheres of government recognized as within the absolute jurisdiction of the king, such as foreign affairs, the army, the navy, the coinage, became more extensive and important in the Tudor period."[14]

Bacon's plans for the reform of natural philosophy, as Martin has argued, played a central role in his commitment to promoting the absolute authority of the monarch. Bacon was one of the most vocal supporters of the divine and absolute rights of the monarch and one of the key strategists in James's quest for legal absolutism.[15] James departed from the Tudor tradition in his attempts to extend the prerogative by establishing legal precedents within the common law for the absolute—as opposed to the "ordinary"—powers of the crown. Bacon's proposals for the reform of the common law, as Martin has suggested, involved selectively culling and compiling those precedents favorable to the expanded power of the king.[16] Justifying the broadest definition of the prerogative within the scope of the common law would, of course, threaten to subordinate the authority of the common law to the authority of the monarch.

Bacon's understanding of the relationship between the king and the common law set him apart from other royal advisers, including his patron Thomas Egerton. Egerton held that the king's prerogative not only was "inheritable & descended from god" but also preceded and was "more auncyente" than either common or statute law; nevertheless, he maintained, "the sovereign was charted to observe the laws that he and his predecessors had created," and he declared in an address to the House of Lords in 1614 that "the King hath no prerogative but that which is warranted by law and the law hath given him." Egerton, moreover, steadfastly protected the "inalienable rights and privileges of the local and regional courts," whose rule, he argued, was grounded in "custom," and "fought royal influence on the behalf of regional authorities."[17] In contrast, Bacon viewed both the regional courts and Parliament with suspicion, asserting that the law rested in the person of the king, Parliament being "more properly a Council to the King, the great Council of the Kingdom, to advise his Majesty of those things of weight and difficulty which concern both the King and Kingdom, than a court." Writing in 1606, Bacon asserted that "The King holdeth not his prerogatives of this King mediately from the law, but immediately from God."[18] For Bacon, the king's will was law.

While in theory both royalists and oppositional parliamentarians held that the king and Parliament were one, the antithetical attempts to expand the reach of the king's prerogative, on the one hand, and the parliamentarians' attempts to protect and expand their authority, on the other, by 1610 posed a dangerous separation between the will of the monarch and that of Parliament. Judson observes that James's counselors and supporters attributed unprecedented scope to the prerogative:

They so exalted the [king's] absolute power that little room was left for the subjects' rights and property, and they so tipped the scales in favor of the prerogative that the old balanced constitution no longer prevailed. They actually extended the monarch's absolute power so far into realms which the law had generally recognized before as belonging to the subject that the law no longer did afford adequate legal protection for his rights and liberty. For these reasons the conception of monarchy which the royalist judges and counselors evolved during these years of controversy was a real departure from the views most men had earlier held.[19]

The arguments advanced by the king's counselors for the expansion of the prerogative were viewed as an immediate threat to both property and liberty. The poet of the *Anniversaries* implicates natural philosophy in its encompassing critique of this absolutist ideology and the threat that it poses to free speech and intellectual freedom. In seeking sanction for the expansion of the prerogative, royalist supporters of legal absolutism, and Bacon in particular, increasingly sought to circumvent common law by grounding their claims in arguments about natural, divine, and national law.[20] As the "law is more worthy than the statute law, so the law of nature is more worthy than them both," argued Bacon in the case of the *post-nati* in 1610. "All national laws whatsoever," Bacon observed, "are to be taken strictly and hardly in any point where they abridge and derogate from the law of nature."[21] While Ellesmere, Coke, and other royalists invoked arguments for allegiance to the king based on natural law, Bacon "presented the most complete and theoretical argument on that basis," suggesting that the absolute authority of the King—and the subject's obedience to that authority—were grounded in the laws of nature, which took precedence and "was never obliterated by later laws." As Judson points out, in the first three decades of the century, parliamentarians grew increasingly suspicious of arguments from natural law, knowing that "if the royalists established their claim that natural law not only reinforced common law, but could, upon occasions determined by the royalists, override it, then the safeguards to property and other rights of the subject provided by the common law would be of no avail."[22] Given the frequency with which arguments from natural law were being raised in Parliament in the debates over the scope of the king's prerogative, Donne and his contemporaries could hardly have understood Bacon's claims to provide an authoritative strategy for interpreting the essential laws of nature as anything other than a means of advancing his political philosophy.

III

In recent years, studies by Annabel Patterson, David Norbrook, Jeanne Shami, and Paul Harland, among others, have challenged and complicated the critical tradition that has seen *Pseudo-Martyr* as marking a crucial transition from the skeptic of the *Songs and Sonets* to the high Anglican apologist for the monarch.[23] Studies by Shami and Harland suggest that the sermons of the dean of St. Paul's may indeed demonstrate a good deal more resistance to James's absolutist claims than critics have previously credited. Shami notes that in engaging, albeit tentatively and discretely, with the political controversies of the period, Donne contrasts to such other prominent divines as Lancelot Andrewes. She suggests, moreover, that Donne frequently invokes the sovereign power of Christ to temper and delimit James's absolutist claims. More immediately relevant to the politics of the poet of the *Anniversaries* period are studies by Patterson and Norbrook, who suggest that in both *Biathanatos* and *Pseudo-Martyr* (1610) Donne continues to register the resistance to the absolutist claims of both pope and king that, as Richard Strier has demonstrated, is so evident in Satire 3.[24]

Marotti has observed that Donne's argument defending the morality of suicide in *Biathanatos* alternately undermines arguments from natural law and attempts to establish a foundation in natural law for the rights of the individual.[25] Donne's resistance to arguments from natural law may also be seen as demonstrating the poet's concern with the role that arguments from natural law were increasingly playing in advancing James's absolutist policies. As Marotti and Strier have both noted, the authority that Donne vests in the individual conscience in *Biathanatos* poses an implicit challenge to the authority of the monarch. In defending the morality of suicide, the poet argues that "obligation which our conscience casts upon us is of stronger hold and of straiter band than the precept of any superior, whether law or person, and is so much *iuris naturalis* as it cannot be infringed nor altered *beneficio divinae indulgentiae.*" The conscience of the individual must, Donne asserts, be the final arbiter of right action. Marotti notes that "Instead of depicting nature as the source of royal authority, [Donne] makes it the basis

of the moral and political autonomy of the individual." Patterson
has argued, moreover, that Donne's assertion in *Biathanatos* that the
"prerogative is incomprehensible, and over-flowes and transcends all
law," may be read as a subversive critique of the prerogative. "To call
the prerogative 'incomprehensible,'" Patterson points out, "is poten-
tially a subversive pun, combining what cannot be understood with
what cannot be contained."[26]

As Patterson has noted, Donne's *Pseudo-Martyr* provides strong
evidence of Donne's sympathy with the parliamentary opposition;
this ostensible defense of the oath of allegiance, she argues, may be
read as subversively delimiting the scope of the king's authority.
Patterson notes that Donne's association with the Mermaid Club
during his years at Mitcham placed him in close contact with
Richard Martin, an outspoken critic of monopolies and James's
absolutist policies, and with Christopher Brooke and John Hoskyns,
vocal champions of "free elections, free speech [and] the liberties of
the subject" in the 1610 Parliament, which distinguished itself by its
opposition to James's attempts to extend the power of the pre-
rogative.[27] In the dedication that prefaces *Pseudo-Martyr*, in fact,
Donne offers a rationale for defending the Oath of Allegiance that
is grounded in a contract theory of government: "Since in prouiding
for your Maiesties securitie, the Oath defends vs, it is reason, that
wee defend it. The strongest Castle that is, cannot defend the
Inhabitants, if they sleepe, or neglect the defence of that, which
defends them." The relationship between monarch and subject is
conditioned upon the monarch's defense of his subjects; the monarch
who persecutes or fails to protect his subjects from persecution,
Donne implies, forfeits the fealty of his subjects. Donne's remarks,
in the same treatise, upon the elevation of the pope to divine status
can equally be read as a critique of the divine and absolute rights of
the monarch: "The farthest mischiefe which by this excesse Princes
could stray into, or subiects suffer, is a deuiation into Tyranny, and
an ordinary ufe of an extraordinary power and prerogatiue, and so

making subiects slaues. . . . But by the magnifying of the Bishoppe of Rome with these Titles, our religion degenerates into super-stition. . . . And therefore to such as claime such a power, it is more dangerous to allow and countenance any such Titles, as participate in any signification of Diuinity."[28]

As Patterson has argued, Donne's critique of the excesses of the papacy in *Pseudo Martyr* may be read as reminding the reader of the dangers of any form of political or theological absolutism. In *The Courtier's Library*, Donne offers acerbic commentaries on sycophants at court and on the absolutist ideology they helped to promote. One entry satirizes one of James's favorites, referring to "Edward Hoby's Afternoon Belchings, or A Treatise of Univocals, as of the King's Prerogative, and Imaginary Monsters, Such as the King's Evil and the French Disease." The association of the prerogative with "Imaginary Monsters" might be seen as suggesting that the power to which James lays claim is both "imaginary" and "monstrous." Donne's disgust for courtiers who advance their own power by advancing the prerogative is also clearly evident in the marginal notations he has scribbled in his copy of *Utopia*, affirming Hyth-loday's critique of the corruptions of court culture with his own references to "cryers up of ye kings prerogative."[29]

IV

While the king and Parliament were embroiled in their dispute over the scope of the king's prerogative, the Jacobean court was absorbing news of an event in the Florentine court of Cosimo de Medici that served as a harbinger of the expanded role that astronomy and natural philosophy would play in the future of statecraft. Galileo's presentation of the *Sidereus nuncius* to Cosimo de Medici in 1610 may have given Bacon new hope for advancement and new cause for concern to Donne and others interested in delimiting the scope of the monarch's power. Galileo's claims in

Sidereus nuncius provided support for Copernicanism, by "contra-
dicting the dominant Aristotelian cosmology" in asserting the
existence of four more planets than the reigning cosmology had
recognized, and in asserting that these four planets "circled Jupiter,
not Earth." As Mario Biagioli has noted, however, of equally
"revolutionary" significance was the authority Galileo claimed in
assigning emblematic significance to his discovery. Galileo presented
the planets to de Medici as emblems of the Medicean dynasty,
reinforcing the authority of their lengthy mythology, which had
long associated the "Cosmos" with "Cosimo" and Jupiter with
Cosimo I, "the founder of the dynasty and the first of the
'Medicean gods'." The Medicean stars, Galileo suggested, provided
celestial—and therefore divine—authorization of the Medicis'
power. Though Cosimo deferred to papal authority in steadfastly
refusing to endorse the literal "truth" of the emblems that Galileo
provided, the prominence he proferred Galileo's findings, and the
speed that marked the astronomer's promotion from mathematician
to philosopher or emblem maker, illustrates, as Biagioli argues, the
role that the court was beginning to play in the "social legitimation
of early modern science."[30] It also serves as an early instance of the
role that early modern science would increasingly play in the
centralization and legitimation of secular political authority.

Galileo's strategy in *Sidereus nuncius* for legitimating his claims
closely resembles the strategy that Bacon adopts in *The Advancement of
Learning*, and both reflect importantly upon the dynamic relation-
ship between the new philosophies and poetry in seventeenth-
century court culture. In what Martin has observed to be a quest
for preferment to the position of court philosopher, Bacon argues
that the power and wisdom of James "deserveth to be expressed not
only in the fame and admiration of the present time, nor in the
history and tradition of the ages succeeding; but also in some solid
work, fixed memorial, and immortal monument, bearing a character
or signature both of the power of a king and the difference and

perfection of such a king."[31] Bacon's natural philosophy will, he
suggests, provide James with the knowledge and material means to
fashion nature into the ultimate emblem of monarchical power, one
which he suggests will outlast any poetic tribute. James—and
Bacon—will be immortalized, their power associated with a legacy
of imperial power drawn from the power of nature.

In his dedication to Cosimo de Medici, Galileo positions his
offering in relationship to, and implicitly in the context of, courtly
competition for the king's favor. In the hierarchy of monuments
that might commend a ruler's name to posterity, Galileo ascribes
greater durability, and thus value, to poetry than to "images
sculpted in marble or cast in bronze." While "the eternal celebration
of the greatest men" is better entrusted "not to marbles and metals
but rather to the care of the Muses and to incorruptible monu-
ments of letters," Galileo suggests that even these works "perish in
the end through violence, weather, or old age." The "ingenuity" and
"dar[ing]" of the astronomer, however, enables him to surpass these
monuments so that "the fame of Jupiter, Mars, Mercury, Hercules,"
and now Cosimo himself "will not be obscured before the splendor
of the stars themselves is extinguished."[32] Biagioli notes that within
the logic of court patronage, to present oneself as having the agency
to proffer the prince any gift, no matter how extraordinary, would
be deemed an offense, particularly since "one could not purport to
present the prince with anything that was not already his." There-
fore, "one could gain legitimation as a scientific author only by
effacing one's individual authorial voice. To be a legitimate author
meant to represent oneself as an 'agent' (maybe a 'prophet') of the
prince." Thus, Galileo purports to be acting not on his own agency,
but on behalf of the "Maker of the Stars himself," who "by clear
arguments, admonished me to call these new planets by the
illustrious name of Your highness before all others."[33] The political
power of the emblems that the astronomer-mathematician turned
court philosopher offered, then, was inseparable from his claim to

be able to interpret the divine order in nature, a claim that the Catholic Church perceived as a threat to its interpretive monopoly over the divine order in nature.

In a letter to James written in 1603, Bacon explicitly asserted that the model for the government of both church and state was to be found in the government of nature, while implicitly presenting his qualifications for the position of court philosopher. William Gilbert, who had served as de facto court philosopher to Elizabeth and whose work advancing his philosophy of the lodestone continued to enjoy currency throughout the century, had recently and rather conveniently followed Elizabeth to the grave. In his letter to the newly crowned monarch, Bacon draws an explicit connection between the government of nature and the government of men:

I do not find it strange (excellent King) that when Heraclitus . . . had set forth a certain book which is now extant, many men took it for a discourse on nature, and many others took it for a treatise of policy and matter of state. . . . And therefore the education and erudition of kings of Persia was in a science which was termed by a name then of great reverence, but now degenerate and taken for an ill part: for the Persian "magic," which was the secret literature of their kings, was an observation of the contemplations of nature and application thereof to a sense politic; taking the fundamental laws of nature, with the branches and passages of them, as an original and first model, whence to take and describe a copy and imitation of government.[34]

Bacon invokes the multiple interpretations sustained by Heraclitus as evidence of an essential connection between state policy and natural philosophy. The quest of Bacon's natural philosophy, the passage suggests, is to locate in nature an incontrovertible foundation for James's absolute authority, and to enable the king to enlarge his power over his subjects by assuming the power over nature that was commonly attributed to the legendary Persian magi.

V

If the claims of Bacon, like those of Galileo, would legitimate secular political authority, they would do so precisely by providing evidence in nature of the divine authorization of the king's power. Far from heralding the arrival of a purely secular approach to nature, Bacon's natural philosophy was framed as a project with explicitly theological motives and implications. In *The Advancement of Learning*, Bacon explicitly and implicitly indicates that his natural philosophy will play a key role in establishing a theological basis for James's claim to an expanded prerogative. "Is not the ground, which Machiavel wisely and largely discourseth concerning governments," Bacon reminds the reader, "that the way to establish and preserve them, is to reduce them *ad principia*, a rule in religion and nature, as well as in civil administration?" Bacon shared with his contemporaries an awareness of the complex relationship among the three branches of philosophy: natural, divine, and civil. The "rule" that Bacon attempts to locate in nature would enable him, in effect, to monopolize all three branches of philosophy. Bacon's natural philosophy, then, would promote and mystify an ideology that seeks to monopolize interpretation and political power.[35]

The goal of Bacon's natural philosophy, as he explicitly asserts in *The Advancement of Learning*, is to provide a definitive reading of the Book of Nature, and this definitive reading is itself synonymous with the project of reconstructing the lost language of Adam. Bacon shared with his contemporaries the belief that language has been implicated along with nature in the fall from grace. In the seventeenth century the inadequacy of human language was seen as reflecting man's fallen moral state and the impairment or loss of Adamic knowledge of God and nature. As Bono has noted, views of the precise nature of Adamic language and of the degree of loss sustained in the fall varied, as did the strategies for the repair—or in Bacon's case, the replication—of this fallen language. In *Valerius terminus* (1603) Bacon specifically indicates that the goal of his reformed philosophical language is the "restitution and reinvesting (in great part) of man to the sovereignty and power (for whensoever he shall be able to call the creatures by their true names he shall again command them) which he had in his first state of creation." Adamic language is, for Bacon, synonymous with knowledge of and control over the constituent elements of creation. While "the perfect, and perfectly *natural* conjunction of words and things Adam experienced in the Garden of Eden has been lost," as Bono and others have noted, Adamic knowledge and language nevertheless serve as the model and ideal for Bacon's reformed natural philosophy and philosophical language.[36]

For Bacon, the replication of the lost knowledge of Adam can be achieved only by abandoning a fallen human language as an instrument for the pursuit of philosophical truth and turning, instead, directly to the Book of Nature. The failure or "error" of scholasticism and of all subsequent systems, Bacon suggests in *The Advancement*, lay in replicating the fallacies that are embedded in language itself. "[F]alse appearances" and implicitly false beliefs, Bacon argues, are "imposed upon us by words, which are framed and applied according to the conceit and capacities of the vulgar sort," and thus do "shoot back upon the understanding of the wisest, and mightily entangle and pervert the judgment."[37] The reform of natural philosophy, then, can only be effected by razing the foundations upon which all previous philosophical systems have been based. Bacon's goal is to bypass and ultimately eliminate the fallacies and suspect ideologies of the "vulgar" that circulate in a fallen language, infecting the body politic.

While the "Sceptics" and "Academics," Bacon observes, mistakenly believed that "the knowledge of man extended only to appearances and probabilities" because of the "deceit" to which the senses were subject, Bacon's inductive philosophy will supply a precise and systematic experimental methodology, that, with the "help of instruments," or prosthetic technologies, will correct the failures and weaknesses of the fallen human senses.[38] As such, Bacon's inductive philosophy would enable the natural philosopher to accurately observe and penetrate to, and ultimately manipulate and control, the "true" nature and underlying "forms" of things presently deemed "too subtile" to be viewed accurately by the senses.

While Bono has argued that Bacon clearly distinguishes between the word of God imprinted in the world of nature and made manifest in Adamic language, on the one hand, and divine will for man as manifested in Scripture, on the other, the distinction is in fact a tenuous one that Bacon alternately invokes and effaces. In *The Advancement of Learning*, he piously concedes that "out of the contemplation of nature, or ground of human knowledges, to induce any verity or persuasion concerning the points of faith, is in my judgment not safe," warning the reader "of the extreme prejudice which both religion and philosophy hath received and may receive by being commixed together; as that which undoubtedly will make an heretical religion and an imaginary and fabulous philosophy."[39]

Bacon also repeatedly indicates, however, that his reading of the Book of Nature will provide a "guide" and a corrective to readings of the Book of Scripture, one that would neutralize scripturally based challenges to the authority of the monarch. Bacon sets out the theological role of his natural philosophy as providing an antidote to skepticism, to "unbelief" and "error":

[L]et it be observed that there be two principal duties and services, besides ornament and illustration, which philosophy and human learning do perform to faith and religion. The one, because they are an effectual inducement to the exaltation of the glory of God: For as the Psalms and other Scriptures do often invite us to consider and magnify the great and wonderful works of God, so if we should rest only in the contemplation of the exterior of them as they first offer themselves to our senses, we should do a like injury unto the majesty of God as if we should judge or construe of the store of some excellent jeweler by that only which is set out toward the street in his shop. The other, because they minister a singular help and preservative against unbelief and error: For our Saviour saith, *You err, not knowing the Scriptures, nor the power of God;* laying before us two books or volumes to study . . . first the Scriptures, revealing the will of God, and then the creatures, expressing his power: whereof the latter is a key unto the former; not only opening our understanding to conceive the true sense of the Scriptures . . . but chiefly opening our belief, in drawing us into due meditation of the omnipotency of God, which is chiefly signed and engraven upon his works.[40]

His program for the reform of natural philosophy, Bacon suggests, will provide a key to the "true sense of the Scriptures," the one literal meaning to which the entire text may be reduced. Bacon's program would, then, eliminate the space for idiosyncratic readings of Scripture and at once erode the authority of the clergy by appropriating the "key" to Scripture for natural philosophy. While Bacon represents natural philosophy here as a meditative practice that enhances one's awareness of the omnipotency of God, his depiction of God as "an excellent jeweler" evokes the material gains that his readings of the Books of Nature and Scripture will assure the king—and himself, as the king's agent—according, of course, to the will of God.

Bacon represents the ancient monarch Salomon (Solomon), with whom James frequently identified himself, as realizing the peculiar role of the monarch as the consummate natural philosopher, the ideal reader of the Book of Nature. In this passage, knowledge of the powers of nature is explicitly associated with material gain:

[I]n the person of Salomon the king, we see the gift or endowment of wisdom and learning. . . . By virtue of [a] grant or donative of God, Salomon became ennabled not only to write those excellent parables or aphorisms concerning divine and moral philosophy, but also to compile a natural history of all verdure, from the cedar upon the mountain to the moss upon the wall . . . and also of all things that breathe or move. . . . Nay, the same Salomon the king, although he excelled in the glory of treasure and magnificent buildings, of shipping and navigation, of service and attendance, of fame and reknown and the like, yet he maketh no claims to any of these glories, but only to the inquisition of truth; for so he saith expressly. *The glory of God is to conceal a thing, but the glory of the king is to find it out;* as if, according to the innocent play of children, the Divine Majesty took delight to hide his works, to the end to have them found out; and as if kings could not obtain a greater honour than to be God's playfellows in that game.[41]

Bacon foregrounds the material benefits that will accrue to the king and empire by understanding and channeling God's power in nature. At the same time, he valorizes the exploitative goals of his natural philosophy, assuring James of the piousness of his project by suggesting that its highest attainment will be insight into divine truth, and by representing the philosopher-king as God's innocuous playfellow in nature. Despite Bacon's assertions to the contrary, the "truths" that would be gleaned from studying the Book of Nature are, for Bacon, consistently identified with insight into the means through which the individual elements of nature can be controlled and manipulated. Control over the elements of nature is synonymous for Bacon with the omnipotence of God, and it is precisely this all-encompassing power that Bacon would ostensibly confer upon James. Immediately following the passage cited above, Bacon elevates Salomon to a status that rivals that of Christ, whose capacity to manipulate nature is, for Bacon, a mark of his divinity:

Neither did the dispensation of God vary in the times after our Saviour came into the world; for our Saviour himself did first shew his power to subdue ignorance, by his conference with the priests and doctors of law, before he shewed his power to subdue nature by his miracles. . . . So in the election of those instruments which it pleased God to use for the plantation of the faith, notwithstanding that at first he did employ persons altogether unlearned otherwise than by inspiration, more evidently to declare his immediate working, and to abase all human wisdom or knowledge; yet nevertheless that counsel of his was no sooner performed, but in the next vicissitude and succession he did send his divine truth into the world waited on with other learnings as with servants or handmaids.[42]

As in his letter to James in 1603, Bacon conflates natural, divine, and national law, implicitly representing himself as uniquely qualified to provide the kind of counsel that, in his account, both licenses and enables Christ's, and implicitly James's, powers to subdue nature, theological error, and in Bacon's encompassing use of the word "ignorance," an evidently broad range of misconceived beliefs. The passage demonstrates Bacon's desire to marginalize the politically subversive implications of the doctrine of the "inner light." Divine truth is, in the present, no longer available by means of "inspiration" to the vulgar and "unlearned" but is the exclusive province of an interpretive elite. Though Bacon generally casts his natural philosophy as an agressively masculinist enterprise, its status as feminized "handmaid" in this passage valorizes it as a passive instrument of a patriarchal God. Bacon's technocratic elite, however, are implicitly masculinized, identified with the apostles and indeed with Christ himself. While Bacon's conception of natural law specifically precludes divine eruptions in the natural order, the experimental strategies of Bacon's new apostles will serve a function similar to the miracles performed by Christ and the apostles, enabling them to "subdue" not simply nature but also skeptical and implicitly political resistance to the authority of God and king.

His encompassing promises to James to provide him with the insights of Salomon, and indeed of Christ himself, are tempered by pious assertions that nature can yield "no perfect knowledge" of God but only "wonder, which is broken knowledge." Elsewhere in

The Advancement, however, Bacon warns against the belief that "a man can search too far or be too well studied in the book of God's word, or in the book of God's works . . . but rather let men endeavor an endless progress in both."[43] The goal toward which this "endless" progress or proficiency is directed is an unassailable reading of the Book of Nature and the disclosure of a "summary" law of nature that is identifiable with perfect knowledge of the divine, underlying order in nature and perfect control over all of creation.

Despite Bacon's "extensive preoccupation with the inadequacies of words," as Robert Stillman observes, Bacon's reformed natural philosophy nevertheless mystifies "the necessary linguistic mediation between the mind and nature." Charles Whitney offers a similar critique, noting that while Bacon attacks Paracelsus and the alchemists for their dependency upon analogies, their belief in specious "correspondences and parallels" that ostensibly link microcosm and macrocosm, the human body and "all varieties of things, as stars, plants and minerals, which are extant in the great world," the taxonomical divisions and classifications through which Bacon would delineate the "forms" and "simple natures" of things are themselves derived by means of analogy. While Bacon's classificatory schema might indeed yield enhanced instrumental capability, the most insidious and unique aspect of Bacon's program for the reform of natural philosophy—and language—is his tendency to deny the agency of the individual interpreter, thereby mystifying "those desires that have led him to organize reality in this way rather than some other."[44]

For all his apparent mistrust of language, Bacon nevertheless gestures in *The Advancement of Learning*, and subsequently in *The Wisedome of the Ancients*, toward the creation of a perfected philosophical language that will serve as the vehicle for the transmission of the underlying truths and univocal "meanings" of the elements of the Book of Nature. As Stillman observes, however, Bacon maintains a "remarkable silence about the kind of discourse required for philosophical communication and the practical necessities that

motivate such discussions as he entertains," and provides "no indi-
cation as to whether it will replace or merely supplement existing
languages." Particularly in *The Advancement of Learning*, Bacon falls back
upon attacking the linguistic practices of existing philosophical
systems, ironically insisting, as Stillman notes, on the virtues of a
"plain style." The "great sophism of all sophisms," Bacon asserts, is
"equivocation or ambiguity of words and phrase, specially of such
words as are most general and intervene in every inquiry."[45] Donne's
equivocal "she," who intervenes at every juncture of the *Anniversaries*,
can be seen as a satirical rejoinder to Bacon's quest for a perfect
philosophical language.

If an accurate and exhaustive reading of the Book of Nature,
associated with the disclosure of the "summary" law, remains a
distant goal for Bacon, the "broken knowledge" or contingent claims
that the natural philosopher would supply would nevertheless be
authorized by their proximity to this ideal, and by the monarch's
institutional licensing of the natural philosopher's monopoly over
the philosophical and technological instruments for interpreting the
Book of Nature. The motivating desire behind Bacon's quest for a
reformed philosophical language, and more broadly, his reformed
natural philosophy, is to reduce the multivalent "meanings" of
things and words and impose a single, literal interpretation upon
the text of nature that would, in turn, govern readings of Scripture
and erect a new foundation for "civil administration." The natural
philosophy and reformed philosophical language that Bacon
envisions would eliminate the space for idiosyncratic interpretation
that is synonymous for Bacon with political dissent and opposition
to the absolute authority of the king.

VI

The reductiveness of Bacon's interpretive methodology is evident
in his *Wisedome of the Ancients*. Bacon's strategy for interpreting the

myths mirrors his project of providing a definitive reading of the
Book of Nature and effectively marginalizing alternative interpreta-
tions to the status of "idols of the mind." Lisa Jardine has observed
that Bacon's interpretive methodology departs distinctly from "the
eclectic and encylopaedic" approaches of Comes and Boccacio, who
"collat[ed] together all available sources which might cast light on
each myth."[46] Bacon, by contrast, presents a single, definitive version
of each myth, minimizing details and omitting previous interpre-
tations inconsistent with the argument of each for the central role
of natural philosophy in the restoration of the wisdom of the
ancients.

Bacon's self-conscious attempts in his preface to distinguish the
"fables" from the indulgences and fictions of mere poetry is
representative of a larger strategy, evident throughout his work, to
establish an unproblematic dichotomy between the real and the
ideal in order to delegitimate alternative representations and
establish his monopoly over "True Philosophy."[47] "I suppose some
are of opinion," writes Bacon, "that my purpose is to write toyes
and trifles, and to usurpe the same liberty in applying, that the
Poets assumed in faining." Bacon's narrowly constructed definition
of poetry contrasts markedly with that of George Puttenham, his
contemporary at court. Puttenham invokes Aristotle's encompassing
definition of the poet as "maker." Puttenham suggests that poets
were the first historiographers and the "first obseuers of all naturall
causes & effects in the things generable and corruptible, and from
thence movnted vp to search after the celestiall courses and
influences, & yet penetrated further to know the diuine essences and
substances separate. . . . They were the first Astronomers and
Philosophists and Metaphysicks." For Puttenham, all arts and disci-
plines have their origins in poetry. The poet is one who mimetically
recreates both human and natural history. Sir Philip Sidney,
however, contrasts the realism of the astronomer and the natural
philosopher with the idealization of the poet. The poet's office

differs markedly from that of the former two, who faithfully report on the natural order. As Sidney argues: "Only the Poet disdaying to be tied to any such subiection, lifted vp with the vigor of his own invention, dooth growe in effect into an other nature: in making things either better than Nature bringeth forth, or, quite anewe, formes such as never were in Nature . . . so as he goeth hand in hand with Nature, not inclosed within the narrow warrant of her guifts, but freely ranging, onely within the Zodiack of his owne wit."[48] Just as the poet may perfect the natural world through his images, making the "too much loued earth more louely," he creates images of human perfection that inspire men to virtuous acts. The historian, by contrast, is tied to reporting only what actually took place and therefore is more likely than the poet to provide models of human behavior that encourage human corruption. Poetry, argues Sidney, is more conducive to the development of human virtue than all other "competitors," the poet therefore having the greater claim to statesman than the practioner of any other art. Sidney's claim for the privileged position of poetry and the poet, then, rests upon a problematic distinction—drawn from Aristotle's poetics—between the real and the ideal, a distinction that Bacon subsequently invokes to undermine the moral and political authority of the poet.

While heralding the capacity of the poet to provide models of virtue, Sidney's *Apologie for Poetrie* also nods toward the role of poetry as a vehicle for responding to the abuse of monarchical power. The *Apologie*, Annabel Patterson argues, "contains a condensed argument about the relationship between literature and sociopolitical experience. If you live 'under hard lords or ravening soldiers,' you may have to communicate 'under the pretty tales of wolves and sheep.'" Puttenham similarly represents the role that poetry has traditionally played as a means of addressing political injustice. He notes that Virgil "deuised the Eglogue . . . not of purpose to counterfait or represent the rusticall manner of loues and communication: but vnder the vaile of homely persons, and in rude speeches to insinuate and glaunce at greater matters, and such as perchance had not bene safe to have beene disclosed in any other sort."[49] Sidney's oft-quoted claim, then, that "The poet nothing affirms and therefore never lyeth," effectively serves to shield the poet from accountability for the political reverberations of his narratives.

Bacon's dismissal of poetry as trivial fictions undoubtedly reflects his recognition of the arena that the cultivated ambiguity of Elizabethan and Jacobean poetry provided for critiques of and challenges to the authority of the crown. His marginalization of poetry in this respect must be seen as part of a Machiavellian strategy to neutralize political threats rather than exacerbating them through direct forms of censorship. In his essay "Of Seditions and Troubles," published in 1625, Bacon argues against the too heavy hand of the censor:

Libels and licentious discourses against the State, when they are frequent and open; and in like sort false news often running up and down to the disadvantage of the State, and hastily embraced, are amongst the signs of troubles. . . . Neither doth it follow, that because these fames are a sign of troubles, that the suppressing of them with too much severity should be a remedy of troubles, for the despising of them times checks them best, and the going about to stop them but make a wonder long-lived.

While, as Patterson has observed, Bacon's concern in this passage "would seem to be more with blatant anti-governmental propaganda, the less 'literary' because the more 'open,'" the more covert subversive messages could be dealt with effectively by simply relegating them to the status of "mere fiction," subordinated to the authorized truths of licensed historical accounts and to the authoritative truths that Bacon's natural philosophy would provide.[50] Bacon's dismissal of poetry as trivial fiction becomes a means of marginalizing the social and political authority of poetic "voluntaries," whose subversive messages might make it past the crown censor, until more effective means can be devised for identifying and regulating dissent.

In *The Advancement of Learning* Bacon implicitly identifies poetic "liberty" as a dangerous political "license": "Poesy is a part of learning in measure of words for the most part restrained, but in all other points extremely licensed, and doth truly refer to the Imagination; which being not tied to the laws of matter, may at pleasure join that which nature hath severed, and sever that which nature hath joined, and so make unlawful matches and divorces of things."[51] Bacon's identification of poetry with the imagination both masks and reveals his concern with the potentially politically subversive role of the poet. The poet, whose imagination is not "tied to the laws of matter," is implicitly defined in contrast to the natural philosopher, who legislates "laws of matter" that endorse the authority of the crown. The word *imagination* itself became identified in the seventeenth century with "voluntaries" or challengers to crown authority. Thus the "unlawful matches" or idiosyncratic metaphors of the poet, which reflect a commitment to interpretive heterogeneity, are demonized because they undermine the laws of nature and the crown.

In order, then, to legitimate his reading of the "fables" of the ancients, Bacon divorces them from association with the promiscuous fictions of the poet and implicitly conflates the "fables" with scripture. "Religion it selfe," he observes, "doth somtimes delight in such vailes and shadowes: so that who so exempts them, seemes in a manner to interdict all commerce betweene things diuine and humane." He goes on to suggest that the "fables" may yield some measure of the lost wisdom of the Golden Age, observing that "under some of the ancient fictions lay couched certain mysteries and Allegories, euen from their first inuention."[52] The "fables," then, are associated both with the authority of scripture and with the secret texts of the ancient magi.

In his insistence that the truths of the "fables" present themselves as self-evident, Bacon enacts the interpretive methodology of his natural philosophy, which the myths are made to endorse. His treatment of the myth of Pan is particularly striking. Bacon claims to be able to pierce the "vailes and shadowes" under which the "truths" of the "fables" lie hidden, dismissing altogether the problems posed by figuration and interpretation. The "fables," he suggests, are, in effect, self-interpreting: "I am perswaded (whether rauished with the reuerence of Antiquity, or because in some Fables I finde such singular proportion betweene the similitude and the thing signified; and such apt and cleare coherence in the very structure of them, and propriety of names wherewith the persons or actors in them are inscribed and intitled) that no man can constantly deny, but this sense was in the Authours intent and meaning when they first inuented them, and that they purposely shadowed it in this sort."[53] Bacon's concern with and confidence in penetrating the "fables" to yield the "Author's intent" parallels his belief in the possibility of distilling the literal meaning of the book of nature—and by implication, Scripture.

In his treatment of the myth of Pan, Pan equates poetry with failed interpretive strategies, which are unable to locate the underlying order of nature and thus are seen as engendering social chaos. Pan, who is identified both with nature and with the processes through which natural order is disclosed, is "reputed" to have a daughter, a "litle Girle called *Iambe*," by a woman also named Iambe. While denying that Pan enjoyed conjugal relations with Iambe, and absolving Pan of any role in the creation of the child Iambe, Bacon goes on to suggest that the "tatling Girle . . . represent[s] those vaine and idle paradoxes concerning the nature of things which haue bene frequent in all ages, and haue filled the world with nouelties, fruitles if you respect the matter, changlings if you respect the kind, sometimes creating pleasure, sometimes tediosnes with their ouermuch pratling."[54] Far from serving any productive moral or political purpose, poetry is depicted as an idle and tedious gossip whose various and varying tales engender skepticism, undermining belief in the capacity of humans to penetrate the natural order and, worse, undermining belief in the existence of that order.

Bacon's natural philosophy, then, identified with the masculine figure of Pan, is set in sharp contrast to the mutable and feminized discourse of poetry, identified with the girl child Iambe. "Pan (as his name imports) represents and layes open the All of things or Nature." In contrast to the treatments of Comes or Boccaccio, who identify Pan with nature alone, Bacon identifies Pan with "discreet observation & experience" or Bacon's own experimental procedures, which will yield "universall knowledge of the things of this world."55

If Pan is identified with both nature and the activities of "observation & experience," his wife, Eccho, is identified with "true philosophy," with the unproblematic representation and transmission of the truths that observation and experience of nature yield: "It is an excellent inuention, that *Pan* or the world is said to make choise of *Eccho* onely (aboue all other speeches or voices) for his wife: for that alone is true philosophy, which doth faithfully render the very words of the world, and is written no otherwise than the world doth dictate, it being nothing els but the image or reflection of it, nor adding any thing of its owne, but only iterates and resounds." The goal of Bacon's experimental program, then, is the attainment of this philosophical ideal, this "true philosophy" that will merely "echo" the divine signatures in nature, providing a verbal "image or reflection" of it, without remainder or ambiguity. Whitney has astutely observed that "Bacon's Echo, the colorless univocity of scientific discourse that merely repeats the voice of nature, provides its own critique by being so pointedly a reduction of previous mythographers' and poets' exploration of this creature's symbolic polyphonies."56 The polyphonic nature and ambiguous "she" whose absence echoes throughout the *Anniversaries*, as I will argue in the next chapter, might be seen as Donne's linguistic and epistemological rejoinder to Bacon's "True Philosophy" and his attack on poetry.

VII

Like the virtuosi of the Royal Society in the latter half of the century, though Bacon purports to locate the divine order inherent in nature as Second Scripture, he also invokes the central role that natural philosophy will play in restoring originary order to the chaos of a corrupt, fallen, and conspicuously feminized natural world. The central role that Bacon's misogynist rhetoric played in shaping an ethic of environmental exploitation that persists today has been explored by historians of science, most notably Carolyn Merchant, Evelyn Fox Keller, and Brian Easlea. Bacon's depictions of nature as a wanton woman whose seductiveness both invites and justifies the sexualized investigation and, ultimately, conquest and containment by the male experimentalist, as Merchant notes, constitutes a marked departure from representations of nature as a benevolent and maternal figure. Maternal representations of nature served to foster an ethic of environmental restraint, barring certain procedures—most notably mining—as acts of violence against "her" body. Such is the view of nature that characterizes Gilbert's *De magnete,* which retained considerable currency throughout much of the seventeenth century. The persistence of the figure of maternal Nature is evident also in the latter half of the century in the writings of Milton and the radicals, among others. The transformation of maternal Nature into a corrupt and sexualized figure, as Merchant notes, encouraged the exploitation of nature resources—particularly in the New World—and the growth of industrialization and capitalism.[57] Bacon's equivocal emphasis on the corruption of nature serves the critical function of justifying the exploitation of natural resources in England and the New World essential for the creation of a British empire.

In his *Aphorisms,* Bacon's division of nature into "species of things," "monsters" and "things artificial" is representative of a rhetorical tradition that justifies the technological appropriation of nature:

Nature exists in three states, and is subject as it were to three kinds of regimen. Either she is free, and develops herself in her own ordinary course; or she is forced out of her proper state by the perverseness and insubordination of matter and the violence of impediments; or she is constrained and moulded by art and human ministry. . . . [i]n things artificial nature takes orders from man, and works under his authority: without man, such things would have never been made. But by the help and ministry of man a new face of bodies, another universe or theatre of things, comes into view.[58]

Without the "ministry" of the pious natural philosopher, feminized nature is forever subject to the "perverseness" and "insubordination" of the base "matter" from which she is indistinguishable. The rhetoric of corruption and redemption fuels Bacon's program of harnessing nature on behalf of a British empire and fashioning it into an emblem of the king's power. Redemption and exploitation are, in fact, one and the same.

The rhetoric and philosophy of torture intersects in Bacon's natural philosophy with the rhetoric of misogyny to justify his ethic of environmental exploitation. In his treatment of the myth of Proteus in *The Wisedome of the Ancients* (1609), Bacon suggests that nature can be brought into a state of order only through natural philosophy, which, in effect, subjects "her" to the rack and the manacle:

If any expert Minister of Nature shall encounter Matter by main force, vexing, and vurging her with intent and purpose to reduce her to nothing; shee contrariwise (seeing annihilation and absolute destruction cannot be effected but by the omnipotency of God) being thus caught in the straites of necessitie, doth change and turn her selfe into diuers strange formes and shapes of things, so that at length (by fetching a circuit, as it were) shee comes to a period, and (if the force continue) betakes her selfe to her former being. The reason of which constreint or binding will bee more facile and expedite, if Matter be laid on by Manacles, that is, by extremities.[59]

The eroticized rhetoric of misogyny that characterizes Bacon's descriptions of the material world serves as an argument for the subjection of nature. As Merchant has observed, Bacon's description of the technological manipulation of nature reverberates with imagery drawn from legalized torture, and from the interrogation of witches in particular.[60] In this passage, nature is depicted as a wanton woman whose resistance to her experimental inquisitor only heightens his voyeuristic pleasure in observing the shape-shifting that culminates in a static state marking her subjection to his sexualized power.

If Bacon insists on the one hand that his definitive reading of the Book of Nature will provide an antidote to scripturally based challenges to the authority of the king, he also represents Nature herself as an unruly subject in need of technological rehabilitation by the natural philosopher acting at the king's behest. Foucault has suggested that the goal of torture is to brand the subject with the power of the state; the goal of Bacon's experimental program, as this passage indicates, is to brand feminized Nature with the power of the monarch—and the experimentalist.[61] Nature, for Bacon, is a recusant subject who must be subjected to a regimen of techno-logical rehabilitation by the natural philosopher acting at the king's behest; only through the intervention of the natural philosopher can Nature be "returned" to her originary state of faithfulness— and subjection—to the authority of God and king.

Bacon's emphasis on the utility and material benefits of natural philosophy, as Lesley B. Cormack has pointed out, is rooted in continental influences beginning to invade England in the early seventeenth century. These influences were reflected most strongly in England in the circle of astronomers, natural philosophers, and mathematicians surrounding Henry, Prince of Wales. By 1610 Henry's court, rather than that of James, was the focus of developments in these fields. Henry's interest in the advancement of technological development, of astronomy, natural philosophy and mathematics, as

Cormack points out, reflected the prince's imperialist ambitions and his concern with "the practical problems of war and overseas expansion."[62] By 1610, then, developments in the New Philosophy in England would have been viewed as potential tools for Henry's quest for Protestant hegemony and, more generally, for nationalist ambitions. The dedication of his 1612 essays to Prince Henry indicates Bacon's awareness of the role that his natural philosophy, with its utilitarian emphasis on the technological development and manipulation of nature, might serve in realizing Henry's ambition of fashioning an international Protestant hegemony.

The prominence of the iconography of Astraea during the festival celebrating the Prince of Wales's coronation in 1610 signaled the imperialist ambitions of the young prince, who would, as William Hunt has noted, "do battle with the great Beast itself, the Anti-Christ of Rome," and "lead the Protestant crusade of which Leicester and Sidney had dreamed." The figure of Astraea, whom Marjorie Hope Nicolson, following Hiram Haydn, numbers among the pantheon of characters embodied in Donne's "she," was by 1610 increasingly associated with the imperialist ambitions of the young prince. In Virgil's Fourth Eclogue, the rule of Astraea or Justice was associated with a prehistoric period of world peace. Astraea was said to have left earth during the fallen Age of Iron, and her return, under the Emperor Augustus, was to hail the return of the Golden Age of Justice made possible by a worldwide empire under the rule of Roman law. The figure of Astraea, Frances Yates observes, informs Dante's idealized Beatrice (a figure to whom Donne's "she" has also been compared) and is reflective of the ideology of his *Monarchia*, a work that Yates terms "the most striking statement of imperialist theory in medieval times."[63]

The iconography of Astraea played an important role in the pageantry surrounding the installation of Henry Stuart as Prince of Wales in June 1610 and reflects his desire to dissociate himself from the iconography and corruption of his father's court. In the celebratory masque *Tethys Festivall*, written by Samuel Daniels, with theatrical designs by Inigo Jones, Henry was presented with the sword of Astraea, the icon with which Elizabeth had frequently been associated.[64] From 1604, the year before Bacon published *The Advancement of Learning*, Henry had already begun to view himself "in the ranks of such Protestant soldiers of Europe as Henry IV . . . and Prince Maurice of Nassau." "Henry's Court," Cormack suggests, "provided an alternative to the corrupt and suspect court of his father, allowing the English to identify Henry with England's heraldic past and encouraging them to think of him as a future imperial conquerer." That Henry's empire would be shaped by his vehement anti-Catholicism is evidenced in the composition of his court, many of whom evinced "strong Protestant or even Puritan leanings."[65] Henry would "permit no Catholics in his household,"[66] and certainly none in his bed, having pledged to wed himself to none but a Protestant princess and empire.

The association of Astraea with the iconography of Prince Henry was not lost on seventeenth-century readers of the *Anniversaries*. Donne's poems, in fact, exerted a strong influence on the elegies that marked the death of the prince in 1612. Donne's appropriation of the iconography of Astraea to commemorate the death of the fifteen-year-old daughter of his would-be patron may nevertheless be read as a subversive gesture; in elevating Elizabeth Drury, Donne may be seen as simultaneously devaluing the authority of the dead queen and prince.[67] The praise that Donne offers the dead prince in his own 1612 elegy to Henry, after all, pales somewhat in comparison to the hyperbolic terms in which Donne commemorates Drury, and the iconography of Astraea is surprisingly absent. If Donne's 1612 elegy to the young prince is, as William Hunt rather slightingly observes, "even by Donne's standards laboured and artificial," the quality of Donne's elegy might be a measure of the poet's ambivalence toward, or even resistance to, Henry's imperialist ambitions. The verse, Hunt observes, recounts the belief of many of his contemporaries that "Henry's rule would establish universal peace throughout Christendom, and that this peace would precipitate the Second Coming and Last Judgement."[68] In fact, the poem focuses not on the peace associated with the millenium, but on the warfare that the millenarian fervor surrounding Henry's court is depicted as engendering, when "In Peace-full times, Rumors of Warrs should rise" (42). The poet's conspicuously unresolved question: "Was His great *Father's* greatest Instrument, / And activ'st spirit to convey and tye / This soule of *Peace* throughout CHRISTIANITIE?" (32–34) might be read as scrutinizing, rather than unambiguously reinforcing, the belief that Henry's extreme Protestantism will serve the goal of creating a unified European kingdom.[69] By 1610 the technologies that Henry's patronage supported, as well as those currently supported by James, were seen as means of accessing and exploiting the natural resources of the New World, and as providing both ideological and material tools for waging a holy war against other European nations and, more ominously, against Catholics and other dissenters in England.

VIII

Immediately following Bacon's indictment for bribery in 1621, Donne preached a sermon at Whitehall in which he used the occasion to attack the personal and political motives underlying Bacon's program for the reform of natural philosophy, channeling his personal bitterness at his own thwarted ambitions into an ideological critique. Donne chastizes Bacon for his attempts to elevate James to the status of a god:

We go not about to condemne, or to correct the civill manner of giving different titles to different ranks of men; but to note the slipperiness of our times, where titles flow into one another, and lose their distinctions; when as the Elements are condensed into one another, ayre condensed into water, and that into earth, so an obsequious flatterer shall condense a yeoman into a worshipfull person, and the Worshipfull into Honorable, and so that which was duly intended for distinction, shall occasion confusion.[70]

The remarks serve at once as a broad indictment of the role that flattery too often plays in the politics of patronage in enabling individuals to rise to offices for which they are morally and socially unfit, and, I believe, as a specific attack on Bacon's role in encouraging James to lay claim to what Donne terms in *Pseudo-Martyr* the "signification of Diuinity." Donne's comments might be seen also as a critique of James, who was notoriously profligate in his dissemination of honors and monopolies; the Dean of St. Paul's, however, demonstrates a politic caution in subsequently deflecting his critique onto Bacon's lesser patrons.

The sermon shows the extraordinary skills at equivocation which appear to have enabled Donne to rise to the deanship of St. Paul's while retaining a measure of the skepticism toward authority that characterizes the poetry of the courtier rake. The Dean of St. Paul's goes on to offer a voluntarist critique of the absolutist goals that underlie Bacon's programs for the reform of natural philosophy and the common law:

Gods ordinary working is by Nature, these causes must produce these effects; and that is his common Law; He goes sometimes above that, by Prerogative, and that is by miracle, and sometimes below that, as by custome, and that is fortune, that contingency; Fortune is as far out of the ordinary way, as miracle; no man knows in Nature, in reason, why such, or such persons grow great; but it falls out so often, as we do not call it a miracle, and therefore rest in the Name of Fortune.[71]

In this passage Donne offers a voluntarist critique of Bacon's natural philosophy, challenging a deterministic conception of natural law that specifically precludes God's miraculous interventions in nature. Donne's comments on the workings of God in nature also reflect analogically on the relationship between the common law, the prerogative, and the regional courts, whose authority was commonly viewed as rooted in ancient "custom," and specifically contest Bacon's construction of the relationship among these three powers. Insofar as Bacon's natural philosophy provides a model for political order, his attempts to codify the absolute power of the monarch within natural law is, Donne suggests, an attempt to *delimit* the authority of the monarch. By suggesting that God works *through* a natural law that is subject both to divine intervention and to other contingencies that, however indirectly, reflect the inscrutable will of God in nature, Donne attempts to preserve a unified model of the body politic in which the courts of the common law are at once extensions of monarchical authority and distinct from it. Donne preserves the authority of the common law and the regional courts by suggesting that their powers are consistent with, and operate by, the authority of the monarch. At the same time, Donne specifically absolves James for responsibility in Bacon's rise and fall, displacing it onto the contingencies of "fortune," and implicitly on lesser patrons such as Egerton, who was, after all, the most vocal proponent of the authority of the regional courts.

Undoubtedly recalling the years in which he struggled unsuccessfully to secure preferment, Donne goes on to reflect on the vagaries of the patronage system that advanced Bacon to power and prominence: "Men have preferment for those parts, which other men, equall to them in the same things, have not, and therefore they doe but find [their offices]; and to things that are found, what is our title? . . . If we restore not that which we finde, it is robbery."[72] In the social semiotics of the postlapsarian world—and especially in the world of the court—status, Donne suggests, is a mark of neither divine election nor inherent worthiness. Titles are slippery signifiers that the individual "finds" but must nevertheless earn by respecting the reciprocal obligations of patronage, which Bacon has ignored in his attempt to monopolize the king's power at the expense of his former patrons. For Donne, the Baconian quest for self-evident truth and for a perfect system of representation can never be realized, and its pursuit is motivated by the desire to usurp the freedom of thought and expression that is central to the art of the still skeptical poet of 1611 and 1612.

For the poet of the *Songs and Sonets*—and, I believe, of the *Anniversaries*—nothing is self-evident; all knowledge claims are subject to continual interpretation and reinterpretation. The *Songs and Sonets* read like rhetorical battlefields on which the speaker attempts to draw competing accounts into question, casting doubt on alternative representations of the world, moral action, and self. The exhortation in Satire 3 (1596) to "Doubt Wisely" is an acknowledgment of the mystery, inexhaustibility, and inescapability of metaphor, which Donne's poetry—characterized by paradox, wit, and irony—embodies. "Doubt Wisely" is also a methodological imperative that, in Donne's estimation, must inform a Protestant ideology and hermeneutics; it is an argument for the endless construction and deconstruction of both text and self in the impossible but necessary quest for the divine on earth.[73]

For Donne, as for Bacon, the inadequacy of human knowledge and language was a result of the original Fall, just as the apparent disorder in nature was variously seen as reflective of an essential chaos brought about by the fall, and as a function of man's postlapsarian inability to penetrate the divine order in nature. Donne is nevertheless himself given to questing after Adamic clarity in his persistent concern with etymology and in his belief that "To know the nature of the thing, look we to the derivation, the extraction, the Origination of the word."[74] His emphasis on origins reflects the impulse he shares with his contemporaries and that informs the project of natural philosophy: to deny the agency of the human interpreter in order to maintain the possibility of an authoritative system of representation that embodies uncontestable meaning.

Bacon's insistence upon man's capacity to restore both the order of nature and the knowledge and language of Adam through his own agency is, however, conspicuously at odds with the tenets of Donne's voluntarist belief in the justification by grace rather than by human agency. For Donne, the pristine Adamic language remains an ideal that paradoxically must be sought but cannot be realized on earth. The imperfection of language and the apparent disorder in nature serve as reminders of man's dependence upon the voluntary infusion of divine grace in the world. Fallen language is a function of man's fallen moral state; because man's moral state is not fully perfect in this life, language cannot be rehabilitated.

In Donne's 1621 sermon at Whitehall, Bacon's improprieties provide an opportunity for the Dean of St. Paul's to explode his project of creating a perfect philosophical instrument and language. Donne observes that:

The world hath ever had levities and inconstancies. The same men that have cryed *Hosanna* are ready to cry *Crucifige*; but as in Iob's Wife, in the same mouth, the same word was ambiguous, (whether it were *blesse God* or *curse God*, out of the word we cannot tell) so are the actions of men so ambiguous, as that we cannot conclude upon them. . . . There hath alwaies beene ambiguity and equivocation in words, but now in actions, and almost every action will admit a diverse sense.[75]

The passage may be read as both preserving the possibility of Bacon's innocence and calling attention to the disparity between his corruption and the appearance of propriety that has characterized his public career. The various interpretations to which Bacon's behavior is subject demonstrate the futility of his attempts to construct a system of representation that will eliminate ambiguity and preclude equivocation. In a postlapsarian world, and particularly within the

corrupt economy of the Jacobean court, the meaning that underlies
the words and actions of even the most virtuous men may be
subject to continual reinterpretation, just as the motives that under-
lie the interpretations brought to bear on those words and actions
never can be known completely. In his sermon Donne undermines
Bacon's strategy for policing the hearts and minds of the king's
subjects by reminding his listeners that language is unstable because,
in a postlapsarian world, humans are invariably unstable texts, whose
motives and meanings are forever in flux.

While Bacon seeks to redeem language, Donne—even as he is
searching for clarity of etymological origins—attributes a redemp-
tive function to the fallenness of language and, by implication, to
nature as well. Donne perceives human speech as evidence of man's
inferiority to God, who, as the poet writes in *Essays in Divinity*, "will
be glorified both in our searching these Mysteries, because it
testifies our livelinesse towards him, and in our not finding him."[76]
The argument for the voluntarism of God allows Donne to
acknowledge the limitations of language and to preserve the possi-
bility of meaning. The Logos bridges the chasm between sign and
signified, but unmediated perception of the Logos is predicated on
both moral purity and election, and the latter can never be assured
during one's existence on earth. One can gain some knowledge by
studying etymology, but Adamic clarity is finally unobtainable.
Perfect language is the province of God.

IX

The "she" of the *Anniversaries* serves in Donne's poetry as an
emblem of resistance to totalizing narratives, of the wisdom of an
epistemology founded on endless doubt, and of poetry itself.[77]
Donne's views of both women and the material world, I argue in
chapter 2, differ substantially from those of Bacon. However, in a
period in which women's speech was widely regarded as unreliable

and women's inconstancy served as a frequent subject of male poets at court, woman must have seemed to Donne a particularly apt metaphor for metaphor.

Recent studies of Donne's *Songs and Sonets* have considerably complicated existing accounts by critics such as A. J. Smith, who argued that for Donne, women are "'mere objects to be tried, enjoyed, and lightly discarded'." Thomas Docherty has suggested that characteristically, in the *Songs and Sonets*, the speaker struggles to achieve a sovereign self and to validate a "masculinist epistemology and ideology" through the domination of a feminine object of desire whose subjectivity is viewed as inherently threatening and destabilizing.[78] Docherty is quite right to suggest that in Donne's poetry, struggles for masculine domination of a feminine other are cast as attempts to legitimate individual claims, and more broadly, epistemologies that are specifically associated with masculine power. However, in identifying the poet with his rakish personae, and moreover, assuming the existence of a unitary "masculinist epistemology and ideology," Docherty overlooks the extent to which, in poems like "The Flea," the rhetorical and epistemological strategies that the speaker uses to achieve domination are frequently cast as logically flawed, politically suspect, and morally questionable—in effect, as parodying and scrutinizing strategies for legitimating masculine power and authority.

More recent analyses of Donne's treatment of gender by Barbara Estrin, Heather Dubrow, Diana Trevino Benet, and Achsah Guibbory have yielded more complex accounts of the poet's treatment of gender, suggesting that amatory relations in Donne's poetry are not easily reducible to binary accounts of conquest and submission. Collectively these accounts demonstrate the wide range of portraits that the poet offers of women and amatory relations. Dubrow observes that in poems such as "The Canonization" Donne resists the "adulatory subservience" of Petrarchism, by elevating the male speaker to the status of the idealized woman. Estrin, following

William Kerrigan, finds numerous examples in Donne's verse of the poet's desire to transcend the "divisive power struggle of Petrarchan idealization" altogether by constructing idealized portraits of mutual love and reciprocal desire. Benet has explored the poet's fascination with the "potential fluidity of gender identities," and Guibbory, who has examined Donne's anti-Petrarchan verse, and in particular his portraits of the grotesque female body, as a reaction against female rule, has more recently turned her attention to verses that, she argues, demonstrate his desire to celebrate and sacralize sexual love.[79]

While for Bacon, sexual desire in woman marks her identification with a corrupt and chaotic natural world, the poet of the *Songs and Sonets*, as Guibbory has noted, is clearly enamored of both sexual desire and the prospect of reciprocation and consummation. "The Extasie," for example, transmutes sexual desire into spiritual union, but it is the foreplay that fascinates Donne and the speaker who insists that "So much pure lovers soules descend / T'affections, and to faculties, / Which sense may reach and apprehend"(65–66). Though the speaker's concern for his own pleasure is evident in his suasive insistence that without consummation, "a great Prince in prison lies" (68), the speaker nevertheless renders the woman an active, if not equal, agent in the complex power negotiations that precede consummation. "Sapho to Philaenis" may be read as a sophisticated exercise in male voyeurism, but the poet clearly identifies with the desire of the speaker, who lingers longingly over "lips, eyes, thighs" (45). Even, I would argue, the poet's scatalogical portrait of the debased female body in "The Comparison" demonstrates the poet's fascination with the body as he perversely hangs on each grotesque detail. If, for the poet, women are air to men's angels, composed of some lesser substance, the difference between the two is not as clearly defined as it is for Bacon. For Donne, in any case, as the speaker of "Aire and Angels" pronounces, "Love must not be, but take a body too" (10), and poems such as "Sapho to Philaenis" and "The Extasie" suggest that Donne's women are not simply objects to be conquered but also actively desiring subjects.[80]

Estrin is correct to observe that Donne characteristically eschews the valorization of absence, which is so integral to the conventions of Petrarchan adulation. The reciprocal and embodied lovers of these amatory verses, however, differ significantly from the absent, dematerialized and unattainable subject/s of Donne's *Anniversaries*. Ironically, the mutability of the central "she" of the poems bears interesting resemblances to Donne's cynical portraits of women's inconstancy in poems such as his song "Goe, and Catch a Falling Star," "Love's Alchymie" and "The Indifferent." While Donne's representations of the resistance and inconstancy of woman are part of the conventional rhetoric of misogyny in the period, and of a cultural commonplace that identifies woman with the mutability of the material world, in these poems it is precisely the indeterminacy and mutability of woman as "other" that fascinates and perplexes the poet. The mutability of woman in these poems, as in the *Anniversaries*, provides an antidote to the reification of representations of the world and self, which are associated for the poet with entrapment and submission to external authority. In "Loves Alchymie," for example, in which woman is conspicuously identified with the world of matter, the speaker counsels his audience, "Hope not for minde in woman; at their best / Sweetness, and wit, they' are but, Mummy, possesst"(23–24). The poem is a cynical commentary on the ephemeral nature of love: "So, lovers dreame a rich and long delight, / But get a winter-seeming summers night" (11–12). It also reflects, however, the poet's fascination with "hidden mystery," with that which cannot be reduced or "known"—with that which cannot be made "mummy." In this context, "knowing" is itself synonymous with an essential transformation of the "object" and reduction of it to mere materiality. The maternal resonance of "mummy" suggests Donne's sense that to know, finally, is to be known, to be entrapped and subjected to the authority of the Other. Similarly, in "The

Indifferent," in which the speaker professes that he "can love any, so she be not true" (9) constancy is identified as "dangerous." "Must I, who came to travail thorow you," he asks, "Grow your fixt subject, because you are true?" (17–18).[81] In the poems on inconstancy—and as I argue in chapter 2, in the *Anniversaries*—to fully possess and subjugate the object of epistemological desire is, for Donne, to become a "fixed subject," to repudiate the play of representation and interpretation that is so central to the poet's art.

The mysterious "she" of Donne's *Anniversaries* is an emblem of the poet's resistance to interpretive strategies identified with Baconian natural philosophy and with its attempts to establish a true philosophy that will create a nation of "fixed Subjects," beholden to the authority of an absolute monarch. The idealized and dematerialized "she" of the *Anniversaries* may also be seen as a rejoinder to the rhetoric of misogyny that Bacon uses to legitimate his program for the reform of a promiscuous and ostensibly chaotic natural world. Donne's "she" is a reminder of the absence of true philosophy from the postlapsarian world, of the role of metaphor in mediating the relationship between man and God, and of the central cultural and political role of poetry. To the Donne of 1611 and 1612, living in a country fraught with sectarian squabbling and with the machinations and conflicting claims of ambitious courtiers with dreams of waging an international Protestant holy war, the flexibility and contingency of verse offers a promise of order or at least the potential for discerning an imperfect intimation of divine perfection. In the *Anniversaries* Donne depicts a world in which conflicting claims about the natural world reflect the political ambitions of their proponents and, as such, are represented as both the cause and proof of man's fallen state and of the absence of "True Philosophy" in the postlapsarian world. The fragmented world that remains is held together only by the poet who acknowledges the absence of "True Philosophy" in a world of political turmoil, death, and illusion.

2

JOHN DONNE'S
ANNIVERSARIES

Poetry and the Advancement of Skepticism

The *Anniversaries* treat the crisis of representation and interpretation as both the cause and effect of the death of the world and as inextricably related to the corruption of the Jacobean court. One of the most striking features of the poems, moreover, is the extent to which the poet implicates his own practice in the corrupt economy of Jacobean court patronage. David Aers and Gunther Kress, Arthur Marotti, and Heather Dubrow, among others, have provided important insights into Donne's coterie verse as it manipulates the rhetorical and social conventions of epideictic verse to undercut and critique patrons and would-be patrons and subvert the power dynamics of the client-patron relationship.[1] Donne's awareness, nevertheless, of the moral and political compromises that he makes in fashioning his verses to patrons and would-be patrons strongly informs his skeptical critique of the New Philosophy and of the role that it would ostensibly play in reinforcing James's claims to divine and absolute power. The ambiguity of the central "she" of the *Anniversaries,* and the hyperbolic rhetoric of praise in which Donne shrouds her, is an important element of his critique of the corruption and flattery at court and of attempts to establish the absolute prerogative of the king through arguments from natural law.

Ben Jonson's putatively outraged response to the poems, his assertion reported by Drummond that he found the poems "profane and full of blasphemies" and Donne's praises for Elizabeth Drury better suited to the Virgin Mary, seems to have been a fairly representative reaction to the poems. Donne's response to Jonson's outrage, his claim that "he had described the Idea of a Woman and not as she was," has met with a variety of interpretations, none of which adequately addresses either the relationship between the epistemological and social chaos that is a central focus of the poem or the poet's perceived violation against both the social decorum governing the client-patron relationship and the legitimate boundaries of epideictic verse.[2]

Edward W. Tayler's comprehensive study of the *Anniversaries* is the most recent and elaborate example of this critical oversight. Tayler seizes upon Donne's comments to Drummond as elucidating the scholastic epistemology that ostensibly structures the poems; his study enshrines an undifferentiated and ahistorical conception of "Virtue" as the essential condition for knowledge in the poems, and specifically for grasping their central conceit, which, he argues, celebrates the transcendent idea of Elizabeth Drury. Scholasticism, I will argue, is no more privileged than the New Philosophy in Donne's poems; both are implicated in the poet's encompassing critique of representations produced within the corrupt economy of the Jacobean court that is itself a microcosm of a fallen world. In the world of the poems, virtue, like truth, is defined primarily by absence, and as such is associated with the ambiguity of a fallen language, and with a positive skepticism that affirms the political and interpretive freedom of the individual.

I

Donne's *Anniversaries*, as Marotti, Dubrow, and Janel Mueller have observed, extend many of the strategies that the poet employs in his encomiastic verse epistles to patrons and would-be patrons.[3] As Marotti suggests, in Donne's numerous verses to Lady Bedford he adopts a poetic persona that is alternately deferential and authoritative. On the one hand, he transmutes her into a "symbol of a transcendent

Virtue" and casts his identity and very existence as entirely con-
tingent upon her own; on the other hand, he represents his idealized
portraits of her as evidence of his own poetic agency and forces
"the polite hyperboles of encomiastic verse to outrageous extremes,
calling attention to the social and moral bases of the currency he
was inflating," thereby calling into question the veracity of his
representations.[4]

In "To the Praise of the Dead and the Anatomy," the poem that
prefaces the "First Anniversary," Joseph Hall self-consciously posi-
tions the poems within the material economy of court patronage,
implicating the culture of patronage, the poet's motives, and the
poems themselves in the corrupt, postlapsarian world that the
poems depict. It is, I believe, significant that Hall, who was best
known as a poet for his satirical verses, had suffered under the
patronage of Drury for several years until he secured the support of
Prince Henry in 1607. His bitterness at Drury's treatment of him is
clear in the autobiographical account that prefaces his *Works*, in
which he describes himself as "Being full of Cold and Distemper in
Drury-Lane."[5] In any case, it is difficult to imagine that Hall's
minimally strained relations with Drury, together with his reputa-
tion as a satirist, did not inform the manner in which the poems
were received at court.

Hall represents Donne, and perhaps himself, as "this Muse"
whose poem stands between complete chaos and perfect order "in
his spirit's stead"—that is, in the absence of "she." In this moral
netherworld, Hall calls attention to the financial motives that impel
both Donne and himself to eulogize Drury:

> O happy maid,
> Thy grace profest all due, where 'tis repayd.
> So these high songs that to thee suited bine,
> Serue but to sound thy makers praise, in thine,
> Which thy deare soule as sweetly sings to him

> Amid the Quire of Saints and Seraphim,
> And as any Angels tongue can sing of thee;
> The subiects differ, tho the skill agree. (33–40)

The assertion that "Thy grace profest all due, where 'tis repayd" points not simply to the divine payment that God offers to the faithful but also to the self-interest that informs all interpretations of the world, particularly within the economy of patronage. Hall may well number himself and Donne among those in the funeral train who "walk in blacks, but not complaine," consoled by hopes that Drury's patronage will more than fully "requite" whatever loss the two join in lamenting. The introduction is, in this respect, an encomium to the "cunning Pencill[s]" of both poets as well as to Donne's capacity to fashion such a riddling and compromising elegy. Hall seems to suggest that the skill the poet displays is comparable to that of Elizabeth Drury's soul singing to God or to that of the entire "Quire of Saints and Seraphim," though the lines can, of course, also be read as suggesting that the hymn sung by the redeemed soul of Elizabeth Drury is comparable now to that sung by all the angels in the heavens. The ambiguous tone of the passage, and the ambiguity that shrouds the identity of the central "she," demonstrate the complexities of negotiating the social semiotics of patronage and court society. In this respect the passage, like the poems in their entirety, undermines the Baconian quest for a static, self-evident system of representation.

In providing space for the reader to reflect upon the financial motives that seem to have impelled both himself and Donne to eulogize Drury's daughter, Hall—and implicitly Donne—strikes a blow at the self-legitimating discourse of patronage. The discourse of patronage, as Mario Biagioli has noted, presents the patron-client relationship as one that is "honour-bound" and voluntary, based on mutual, if unequal, respect and affection, rather than dictated by economic motives. Patronage, as Biagoli has observed, "was a voluntary act only in the sense that by not engaging in it one would commit social suicide."[6] The *Anniversaries*, like his illicit marriage to Anne More, reveal the poet's profound ambivalence about the compromises involved in advancing within court culture, and his willingness to toy with social suicide. If Donne cannot escape the economy of court patronage and its demands that one deify and canonize one's patrons, at least figuratively, he is apparently incapable of resisting the urge to demystify and satirize the market forces that shape and legitimate truth claims within the economy of court patronage.

Authoritative readings of the natural world are, moreover, prominently implicated in Donne's critique of the economy of patronage. The metaphor of the two books, the Book of Nature and the Book of Scripture, is a constitutive element of the *Anniversaries*, which demonstrate the complex relationship among Protestant theology, science, and models of government. The postlapsarian chaos that the *Anniversaries* depict reflects, in one sense, seventeenth-century contentions over the nature of the physical world and over scriptural interpretation and the politicized struggle for control over both. Donne's description in the *Essays in Divinity* (1614) of the fracturing of the biblical text in the hands of disputatious theologians mirrors the physical chaos depicted in the *Anniversaries:* "So do they demolish God's fairest Temple, his Word, which pick out such stones and deface the integrity of it, so much as neither that which they take nor that which they leave, is the word of God."[7] In the *Essays in Divinity* Donne sees scriptural language as subject to coercive misprision by individuals who construct God's will to justify their own morally and politically suspect ends. In the *Anniversaries* Donne explores the disputes over the nature of the physical world as they extend the seventeenth-century debates over scriptural interpretation. And he indicts, in particular, the strategies of self-serving courtiers for transforming the text of the world into an argument for the absolute power of the highest patron in the land.

II

The identity of Donne's elusive "she" has engendered endless
critical debate, beginning with the speculations of Jonson and
Donne's contemporaries at court.[8] Nicolson, in particular, has argued
that the *Anniversaries* may be read at least in part as a retrospective
tribute to Elizabeth I. The poems assuredly do beg to be read as a
commentary on the reign of the late queen; however, I do not
believe that they are, in this respect, elegies. Nicolson has noted that
Donne "had not been among the poets who in 1603 joined in the
chorus of lament for the dead queen."[9] She argues, however, that
after seven years under the inept and corrupt rule of James I,
Donne looks back nostalgically upon the reign of the Virgin Queen,
whom he had satirized during her lifetime, and offers his apologia.
The poet's comments upon the *Anniversaries* as reported by
Drummond, however, encourage the reader to view Donne's repre-
sentations of Elizabeth I more skeptically. While the poet's claim
that he "described the Idea of a Woman, and not as she was," seems
fairly innocuous and straightforward when applied to Elizabeth
Drury, the force of the remark, as applied to Elizabeth I, undercuts
the poet's praise of the dead monarch. The comment suggests that,
whatever his grievances against the state of England in 1611 and 1612,
they had not effaced his memories of the injustices he experienced
and witnessed under the reign of Elizabeth. Nicolson herself notes
that Donne's own title for the "Second Anniversary," "Of the
Progres of the Soule," was appropriated from his earlier, unfinished
satire of 1601 implicitly commenting upon Elizabeth's claim to
leadership of the Church of England.

Particularly relevant to this discussion is Achsah Guibbory's
argument that Donne's portraits of the grotesque female body in
verses such as "The Comparison" and "Elegy 2: The Anagram,"
both written in the 1590s, may be read as expressions of contempt
for the aging queen who encouraged male courtiers to express their

adulation—and, implicitly, their pleas for preferment—within the conventions of courtly love. The evidence that Guibbory offers, however, of the poet's "unease at submission to female ruler," might as easily be seen as expressions of resistance to the monarchy itself. It was, after all, during the period of antifeminist backlash following the death of the queen, whose rule was seen as a threat to patriarchal order, that Donne composed the companion poems that may be read as the poet's most extreme exercise in the Petrarchan conventions of idealization and lamentation over the loss of the beloved. It is not, however, the queen herself that the poems celebrate, but her *absence*. Insofar as the poems also invite the more conventional reading, they may be seen as elevating the status of the dead queen for the express purpose of subverting the authority of the reigning monarch.

The political implications of Nicolson's argument for including the figure of Astraea in the pantheon of personae embodied by Donne's "she" has been largely overlooked by critics.[10] As I noted in the previous chapter, Astraea was associated in 1610 with the imperialist ambitions of Prince Henry. Astraea's absence from—or shadowy presence in—the poems might well have been seen as anticipating the moment when the Prince of Wales, who consciously associated himself with Elizabeth and the Tudor lineage, would ascend to the throne and restore justice to the realm. At the same time, however, the poems in no way anticipate the return of the absent "she" or, implicitly, the accession of the young prince, nor is the fragmentation associated with the absence of the central figure represented as an entirely negative phenomenon. Rather, the absence of "she" is depicted as opening up a creative space for the poet, who sets out to revive only some semblance of her.

Astraea was associated with the imposition of Roman law. Her absence from the world of the poems may signal Donne's rejection of attempts to transform the common law into a version of Roman law. The absence of Roman law, then, may be seen as liberating; the continual process of interpretation and reinterpretation that is necessitated by the absence of Astraea from the world of the poems may be seen as akin to the ongoing interpretation and articulation of the common law. There can be little question, in any case, as Patterson has recently begun to explore, that the *Anniversaries* are concerned with the scope of the king's prerogative, a point to which I will return.

Though Marius Bewley, for one, has argued that the poems are a cryptic encomium to the Catholic Church,[11] her shadowy presence in the poem ought, I believe, to be seen as undermining claims by both the Catholic and—under the leadership of James—Anglican churches to divine truth. Like *Pseudo-Martyr*, the poems may be read as satirizing attempts to elevate a temporal monarch to the status of God. By emphasizing the absence of the "she" who unites temporal political power and divine truth, the poems undercut the absolutist claims of James, and of both the Anglican and Catholic churches, and of any singular individual or institution purporting to bring about the perfect rule of God on earth.

While acknowledging that the identity of the central "she" of the poems is ultimately irreducible to any single referent, I wish to add one more to the pantheon of figures that reverberate in Donne's ambiguous "she." The myth of Pan, or nature, Bacon remarks in *The Wisedome of the Ancients*, has sometimes been referred to by the name of Penelope; this sort of inaccuracy is, he observes, "a thing very frequent amongst [writers], when they apply old fictions to yong persons and names, and that many tymes absurdly and indiscreetly: as may be seene heere; for Pan being one of the ancient Gods was long before the tyme of *Vlisses* and *Penelope*."[12] It is possible to read Elizabeth as Donne's own Penelope, that "yong" person whose name is applied to a number of "olde fictions" in a manner that Donne recognizes will be construed by many as both absurd and indiscrete. One of the "old fictions" to which Drury's name seems to be applied in the *Anniversaries* is that of the character of Pan's wife, Eccho, whom Bacon associates with his own "True Philosophy."

In a recent study, Dubrow examines the "bodiless Echo" as a conventional trope of Petrarchism and its counterdiscourses, one that is more broadly representative of the internal contestation that ostensibly conventionally Petrarchan verses frequently encode to the agency and veracity of the masculine speaker. While the *Anniversaries* are hardly classifiable as amatory verses, the adulatory stance and the focus on the "death of the beloved" are both characteristic features of Petrarchan verse.[13] Dubrow's argument is particularly significant in light of studies by Marotti and others who have read amatory relations in Petrarchan verse as mirroring the power dynamics of the client-patron relationship. Dubrow's study provides a more complex account of the gendered dynamics of Petrarchism than previous studies, which have alternately emphasized either the disempowerment of the male suitor or, in more recent feminist accounts, the erasure and silence of the woman, who is reduced to an idealized object of masculine desire.

Dubrow argues, in fact, that one of the defining features of Petrarchism is the breakdown of the binary categories of masculinity and femininity.[14] The *Anniversaries* also enact this "elision of gender"; Donne's "she" is the feminine agent through which the poet undermines the hierarchical relationship of patron and client, monarch and subject, and interrogates the social conditions through which masculine speech is authorized.

While, as Dubrow observes, the female voice in Petrarchism can stand for any unruly subordinate discourse, the myth of Echo, she suggests, is frequently associated with the subversive speech of the male poet: "When Echo speaks words that poets themselves might hesitate to utter, the myth allows them again to practice strategies of deflection: they devise yet another plot for excusing their own hostility, attributing it to a voice that is explicitly or, given the myth, at least implicitly female."[15] Bacon's treatment of the myth of Pan, as I have suggested, is a fantasy of reforming and disciplining a promiscuous and implicitly feminine language, and forcing it to utter only the univocal "truths" of the natural philosopher and his patron, the king. For Donne, however, the metaphorical ambiguity associated with unruly feminine speech is the necessary condition for, and agent of, the empowering and subversive speech of the poet. Donne's "she" is a hollow and resounding echo that contests authoritative claims to truth while it celebrates the poet's mastery of the fine art of equivocation, an art that enables him simultaneously to pay self-interested fealty to patron and monarch while engaging in a pious meditation on the absence of divine truth in the corrupt economy of the Jacobean court.

III

While the central premise of the *Anniversaries*, the death of the world, is a common convention of Donne's day, both the extent to which Donne implicates natural philosophy in the sickness of the world and the role that the poet assigns poetry as physic are original. In this respect, the premise of the poems invites the reader to read them as a critique of Bacon's interpretation of ancient myths, his promotion of natural philosophy, and his attacks on poetry. The absence of "True Philosophy" echoes throughout the world of the *Anniversaries*, reflected in the conflicting claims about the nature of man and the world, claims that are represented as themselves engendering chaos in nature and human government. The elusive "she" of the *Anniversaries* can be seen as an emblem of resistance to authoritative claims to truth, and as a reminder of the limitations of human understanding before divine truth. The poet offers the contingent, limited truth of his poetry as an alternative to coercive epistemologies that are the manifestations of a fallen world:

> For there's a kind of world remaining still
> Though shee which did inanimate and fill
> The world, be gone, yet in this last long night,

> Her Ghost doth walke; that is, a glimmering light,
> A faint weake loue of vertue and of good
> Reflects from her, on them which vnderstood
> Her worth; And though she haue shut in all day,
> The twi-light of her memory doth stay;
> Which, from the carcasse of the old world, free,
> Creates a new world; and new creatures be
> Produc'd: The matter and the stuffe of this,
> Her virtue, and the forme our practise is.[16]

The death of the world is here depicted as liberating for the central character because it forces the reader to acknowledge the limitations of human representations in the face of divine mystery and power. The central concern or "matter" of Donne's poem—and ideally of all human creation—is the quest to realize some semblance of divine truth and virtue. The following line acknowledges both that Donne's own art—and ideally all acts of human creation—are attempts to create "forms" of this divine virtue, but "forms" that nevertheless are conspicuously human and subject to continual revision and "practice." Authoritative claims to truth, the attempts of the new philosophers to embody divine truth and virtue, and the political absolutism these claims support are worse than the prattling and tedious tales of the least poet. They reflect an inability to understand the "worth" of divine truth and the limits of human understanding.

In the lines that follow, Donne suggests that insofar as poetry resists authoritative claims to truth and serves as a reminder of the contingency of human understanding, it helps to maintain sociopolitical order. Poetry, like Donne's "she," inoculates the reader against

> hom-borne intrinsique harme,
> (For all assum'd vnto this Dignitee,

> So many weedlesse Paradises bee,
> Which of themselues produce no venemous sinne,
> Except some forraine Serpent bring it in)
> Yet, because outward stormes the strongest breake,
> And strength it selfe by confidence growes weake,
> This new world may be safer, being told
> The dangers and diseases of the old. (FA 80–88)

The most immediate threat to England's nationhood, the lines suggest, comes not from some "foreign serpent" but from an absolutist ideology that erodes individual freedom, even as it fuels the kind of mindset that produces England's quest for an international hegemony. Donne's assertion that "strength by confidence grows weak," moreover, warns his countrymen that smugness produces sociopolitical as well as moral weakness. The lines also serve as a reminder of the tenuousness of status within court culture and suggest that, paradoxically, all real knowledge and power must be grounded in a recognition of the impotence of man before God.

Throughout the poems, Donne undermines authoritative claims to truth. He does so, however, not by directly refuting authoritative claims; rather, by laying on multiple and conflicting claims, he undermines the veracity of all.[17] In this respect, the *Anniversaries* employ a methodological skepticism that bears a significant resemblance to that which Montaigne prescribes in his critique of natural theology, his *Apology of Raymond Sebond*. Montaigne cautions against directly refuting claims; a true skepticism, he suggests, demands even the suspension of disbelief, for "to condemn anything so positively as false and impossible is to claim that our own brains have the privilege of knowing the bounds and limits of God's will, and of our mother nature's power. I have learned too that there is no more patent folly in the world than to reduce these things to the measure of our own power and capacity." Montaigne condemns the claims that "nothing is certaine but uncertaintie," and the assertion that "the Nature of things is but a false and vaine shadow," reflecting that "this manner of speech in a Christian, is full of indiscretion and irreverence; God cannot dye, God cannot gaine-say himselfe, God cannot doe this or that. I cannot allow a man should be so bound by God's heavenly power under the Lawes of our word." Even the Pyrrhonists, Montaigne observes, could not escape from embroiling themselves in contention. What they needed, he noted, was a "new language," for "ours is altogether composed of affirmative propositions, which are directly against them. So that, when they say I doubt, you have them fast by the throat, to make them avow, that at least you are assured and know, that they doubt."[18]

The *Anniversaries* avoid embroiling the poet in the chaos of contrary assertions to which even the Pyrrhonists succumbed. In absorbing the absolutist claims of Baconian experimentalism and the new astronomers into his sophisticated poetic critique of philosophical and political absolutism, Donne demonstrates that poetry, which acknowledges the contingency of all representations, is in fact the highest form of philosophy. Donne's own poetic practice, then, becomes a model hermeneutic, an approach to interpretation and representation that is consistent with a voluntarist theology and a skeptical fideism.

Donne's methodological skepticism is reflected in his treatment of the myth of the Golden Age, which Bacon's natural philosophy seeks to restore. In keeping with his methodological skepticism, Donne does not explicitly reject the myth of the Golden Age but ironically echoes and mimics the lamentations over the lost Golden Age in order to reveal the myth as symptomatic of the human arrogance that brought about the Fall and continues to engender political chaos:

> There is not now that mankinde, which was then,
> When as the Sunne, and man, did seeme to striue,
> (Ioynt tenants of the world) who should suruiue. . . .

When, if a slow-pac'd starre had stolne away
From the obseruers marking, he might stay
Two or three hundred yeares to see't againe,
Then make vp his obseruation plaine . . .
So spacious and large, that euery soule
Did a faire Kingdome and large Realme controule:
And when the very stature thus erect,
Did that soule a good way towards Heauen direct.
Where is this mankind now? who liues to age,
Fit to be made *Methusalem* his page? (FA 112–14,117–20,123–28)

Donne's hyperbolic hymn to the extraordinary physical stature and intellectual capabilities of originary man satirizes the rhetoric of the Golden Age and, implicitly, faith in the human capacity to effect its restoration. The myth of the Golden Age is no more credible than the belief that "an Elephant, or Whale / That met" this mythical man "would not hastily assaile / A thing so equall to him" (139–41). The belief that man was once such a godlike creature simply provides evidence that the prononents of the myth are afflicted with a postlapsarian egoism as well as an insatiable desire for power. They are either gullible enough to believe that "The Fayries, and the Pigmies well may pass / As credible" (142–43), or they imagine everyone else to be so.

Donne goes on to link the myth of the Golden Age to the role that the New Philosophy purports to play in the recovery of lost perfection. The belief that "w'are not retir'd, but dampt" (151) and can restore by our own efforts the lost age of originary perfection underpins the quest for "new phisicke." The "phisicke" of the New Philosophy, Donne suggests, is a "worse Engin farre"(160), which will not only replicate original order but "God's whole worke undue" (155). Donne's reference to the New Philosophy as an "engine" mocks faith in technological progress while playing on the Elizabethan association of "engine" with its Latin root "ingenium," meaning "artifice, trickery, [or] plot."[19] Donne implicitly links the "new physic" with the instruments of warfare or "worse engines" that the new technology will develop.

Donne's equivocal estimations of man in the lines that immediately follow counter Bacon's claims to restore originary order by human agency and emphasize man's dependence on divine grace alone. Donne echoes Montaigne's critique, absorbed from Erasmus, of the arrogance that underlies man's confidence in his privileged position within a natural hierarchy:

> Thus man, this worlds Vice-Emperor, in whom
> All faculties, all graces are at home;
> And if in other Creatures they appeare,
> They're but mans ministers, and Legats there,
> To worke on their rebellions, and reduce
> Them to Ciuility, and to mans vse.
> This man, whom God did wooe, and loth t'attend
> Till man came vp, did downe to man descend,
> This man, so great, that all that is, is his,
> Oh what a trifle, and a poore thing he is! (FA 161–70)

The tone of the passage, like that of the poems taken in their entirety, is ambiguous, and this ambiguity itself underscores the uncertainty of man's position within the natural hierarchy. Donne, like Montaigne, suggests that whatever privileged position man occupies in the universe is not by virtue of his inherent superiority but is dependent upon divine grace and on man's willingness to serve divine God. The God who voluntarily humbles himself to "woo" and serve man provides the model of the just king who uses his power for the benefit of his people and remembers his own dependency upon God. For Donne, as well as Montaigne, the characteristics that most distinguish man from other creatures are his vanity and ambition, which lead him only to defy God and thus reduce man to less than an animal. Invoking scripture, Montaigne suggests that "man . . . is nothing if he but thinke to be something."[20] For Donne, "man by confidence grows weak"; the individual who presumes upon his own knowledge, elevating it to the status of divine truth, becomes nothing but a "trifle, a poor thing."

IV

The most famous lines of the *Anniversaries* have been read historically as invoking the birth of a cultural revolution engendered by the New Philosophy that calls into doubt every aspect of an ostensibly stable, theocentric worldview:

> And new philosophy cals all in doubt,
> The Element of fire is quite put out;
> The Sunne is lost, and th'earth, and no mans wit
> Can well direct him, where to look for it. (FA 205–8)

Far from suggesting that the New Philosophy deliberately challenges a theocentric worldview, these lines recognize that ongoing attempts, whether by the scholastics or the New Philosophers, to undergird theological belief through arguments from the natural order breed skepticism as one paradigm succeeds another. The lines acknowledge also the limitation of any single human interpretation in the face of divine mystery and make ignorance an article of faith. As Charles Coffin suggests, the doubt born of competing interpretation is transformed in the course of the poem into a vehicle for a religion founded on faith. In this respect, the passage is also a riddling allusion to the project of the poem itself, which embodies an interpretive process. If the lines acknowledge the limitations of human intelligence in the face of divine mystery, they also suggest that Donne is the "wit" whose poem demonstrates the new interpretive center. In enacting a noncoercive hermeneutic, Donne's poem provides a new "element of fire" to replace the old ones, which insofar as they are identified with and dependent upon elements in the material world, are so easily snuffed out.

At the same time, however, the lines may well have been read as invoking and satirizing the ostensibly central role of doubt in Bacon's natural philosophy, conflating Bacon's experimentalism with the Pyrrhonic skepticism that Bacon sets out to cure. Within Bacon's experimental program, the role of doubt is specifically limited. The rhetorical emphasis that Bacon places upon doubt in his theory plays a central role in assuring his readers of the legitimacy of his claims. Doubt, Bacon asserts, mediates against the premature forma-tion of systems, which, as he argues, is the downfall of scholasticism and, more recently, of Gilbert's philosophy of the lodestone. Doubt "saveth philosophy from errors and falsehoods; when that which is not fully appearing is not collected into assertion." Similarly, doubt may cause more attention to be paid to items that otherwise have gone unnoticed, except that "by suggestion and solicitation of doubts [it] is made to be attended and applied." If doubt exercises a positive role in encouraging challenges to scholasticism and in the progress toward "true" knowledge of the natural world, the "delivery of sciences" is characterized by a "sparing" use of "confutation" and should "serve to remove strong preoccupations and prejudgements, and not to minister and excite disputations and doubts."[21] The doubt that Bacon directs against "strong preoccupations and prejudge-ments"—which are frequently associated with rival practices and theoretical constructs—also serves the crucial function of reassuring the reader of the accuracy and truth of Bacon's experimental program.

Donne's introduction of the New Philosophy is immediately followed by a passage that links the chaos of competing interpre-tations of nature to the struggle for position within the court:

> When in the Planets, and the Firmament
> They seeke so many new; they see that this

> Is crumbled out againe to his Atomis.
> 'Tis all in pieces, all cohaerence gone;
> All iust supply and all Relation
> Prince, Subject, Father, Sonne, are things forgot,
> For euery man alone thinkes he hath got
> To be a Phoenix. (FA 210–17)

In this passage the atomism that Bacon propounds in the myth of Cupid in *The Wisedome of the Ancients* becomes an image of both celestial and social corruption. Donne's choice of atomism as an image of celestial corruption must be read as a particularly ironic gesture, since the idea of celestial corruption was resisted by the major proponents of the New Philosophy. Donne points to the struggle for a monopoly over the interpretation of nature in his observation that "euery man alone thinkes he hath got / To be a phoenix, and that there can bee / None of that kinde, of which he is, but he." The image, then, represents the New Philosophy as both cause and symptom of the struggle for political authority and individual self-seeking at court.

The incorporation in the subsequent lines of a lengthy conceit, which clearly refers to Gilbert's *De magnete*, extends Donne's exploration of the role that court politics play in legitimating claims about the natural world:

> This is the worlds condition now, and now
> She that should all parts to reunion bow,
> She that had all Magnetique force alone,
> To draw, and fasten sundred parts in one;
> She whom wise nature had inuented then
> When she obseru'd that euery sort of men
> Did in their voyage in this worlds Sea stray,
> And needed a new compasse to find their way;
> Shee that was best, and first originall

Of all faire copies; and the generall
Steward to Fate; shee whose rich eyes, and brest,
Guilt the West Indies, and perfum'd the East;
Whose hauing breath'd in this world, did bestow
Spice on those isles, and bad them still smell so,
And that rich Indie which doth gold interre,
Is but as single money, and coyn'd from her:
She to whom this world must it selfe refer,
As Suburbs and a Microcosme of her,
Shee, shee is dead. (FA 219–37).

The lines provide an ironic commentary on Bacon's dismissal of Gilbert's theory representing the earth as a feminized lodestone. In his indictment of philosophers who "have withdrawn themselves too much from the contemplation of nature, and the observation of nature, and the observation of experience, and have tumbled up and down in their own reason and conceits," Bacon attacks the alchemists who "made a philosophy out of a few experiments with a furnace" and pointedly singles out for humiliation "Gilbertus, our countryman, [who] hath made a philosophy out of the observations of a loadstone."[22] Donne's conceit implicates Bacon's attack on Gilbert as part of a strategy for securing his own privileged position as court philosopher, and implicitly identifies his natural philosophy with the divisive effects of James's absolutist ideology.

In fact, the sequence of the lines beginning with Donne's introduction of the New Philosophy and ending with the conceit based on *De magnete* bears significant similarities to the order of Bacon's discussion in *The Advancement of Learning*. The parallel lends further support to my claim that Donne is responding specifically to Bacon's natural philosophy as representative of the broader role that natural philosophy and astronomy may serve in legitimating Jacobean absolutism. In *The Advancement of Learning* Bacon follows his claim to restore the lost wisdom of the ancients with his attack on the premature formation of systems and on Gilbert in particular. He then reflects on the ostensibly unique role of doubt in his own system, asserting that "if a man will begin with certainties, he shall end in doubts; but if he will be content to begin with doubts, he shall end in certainties."[23]

Donne, however, renders Bacon's absolutist natural philosophy as both cause and result of man's fall from grace into doubt—into both social and epistemological chaos. Donne launches almost immediately into a passage that echoes Bacon's critique of the attempts of astronomers to replicate mathematically the divine order in nature. In Donne's version, however, he implicitly indicts the hubris of both natural philosophers and astronomers as challenging the omnipotence of God by constituting in their own imaginations the divine order they purport to locate in nature:

Hence it cometh, that the mathematicians cannot satify themselves, except they reduce the motions of the celestial bodies to perfect circles, rejecting spiral lines, and laboring to be discharged of eccentrics. Hence it cometh, that whereas there are many things in nature as it were *monodica, sui juris;* yet the cogitations of man do feign unto themselves relatives, parallels, and conjugates, whereas no such thing is; as they have feigned an element of Fire, to keep square with Earth, Water and Air, and the like; nay, it is not credible, till it be opened, what a number of fictions and fancies, the similitude of human actions and arts, together with the making of man *communis mensura,* have brought into Natural Philosophy.[24]

Donne represents poetically Bacon's critique of the arrogance of imposing human aesthetics upon God. Donne's, however, implicates Bacon in his own critique. Conflating astronomy and astrology (which Bacon numbers among poetic fictions) and, implicitly, natural philosophy, the poet represents them as participants in a celestial drama in which the object is to entrap and systematize God:

> They haue empayld within a Zodiake
> The freeborne Sunne, and keepe twelue signs awake
> To watch his steps; the Goat and Crabbe controule,
> And fright him back, who els to eyther Pole
> (Did not these Tropiques fetter him) might runne:
> For his course is not round; nor can the Sunne
> Perfit a Circle, or maintaine his way
> One inche direct; but where he rose to day
> He comes no more, but with a cousening line,
> Steales by that point, and so is Serpentine:
> And seeming weary with his reeling thus,
> He means to sleep, being now falne nearer vs. (FA 263–74)

In the passage, the twelve signs of the zodiac are personified as twelve astronomer-apostles in a scene that is modeled on Judas's betrayal of Christ in the Garden of Gethsemane. The passage critiques attempts to buttress theology with claims about the natural order, representing these strategies as attempts to control God. Bacon, with his vision of the natural philosopher as the "new apostle," is guilty of the spiritual and intellectual hubris he attacks in astronomers.

If Bacon indicts earlier systems of natural philosophy and astronomy for trying to subject God to human understanding, he nevertheless believes that careful attention to the particular elements of nature, systematically culled, can result in true knowledge of the natural world and of God's design within it. For Donne, however, any attempt to limit God to a particular model of cosmological order will only contribute to the chaos engendered by the succession of competing representations of divine order. By making God's perfection—and social order—contingent on belief in a particular model of the physical world, the scholastics created the condition for the social, physical, and theological chaos that the decentered and ostensibly chaotic world of the new astronomy can be made to

represent. The Ptolemaic model, Copernicanism, and Bacon's experi-
mental philosophy are all types, for Donne, of the tower of Babel:

> They who did labour Babels tower t'erect,
> Might haue considered, that for that effect,
> All this whole solid Earth could not allow
> Nor furnish forth Materials enow;
> And that this Center, to raise such a place
> Was far to little, to haue beene the Base;
> No more affoords this world, foundatione
> To erect true ioye, were all the meanes in one.
> But as the Heathen made them seuerall gods,
> Of all the Gods Benefits, and all his Rods,
> (For as the Wine, and Corne, and Onions are
> Gods vnto them, so Agues bee, and war)
> And as by changing that whole precious Gold
> To such small copper coynes, they lost the old,
> And lost their onely God, who euer must
> Be sought alone, and not in such a thrust. (SA 417–32)

Donne's concern here is not with attacking the Ptolemaic universe—
to do so would be to assume, as Montaigne points out, his own
privileged insight into the divine order in nature. Rather, the poet
asserts that the earth, as a measure of human perfection and divine
order, like the human subject that measures it, is fundamentally
incapable of yielding the true and complete knowledge of God that
philosophers continually invoke in their created systems. The
distinctions among the Ptolemaic, Copernican, and Baconian world-
views are collapsed insofar as all are attempts to unproblematically
represent the order of the physical and metaphysical universe and all
conflate limited human perceptions of the material world with
divine truth. In this respect, they disrupt the relationship between
God and man and become catalysts in a process of reverse alchemy

in which the mystical vision of God in the world is shattered into mundane particulars. The passage critiques the material interests that shape the claims of natural philosophers and astronomers within the economy of court patronage and indicts the patently materialistic ends that Bacon's interpretation and rehabilitation of the Book of Nature would serve. His emphasis on observing and manipulating the individual elements of nature is equated to the pursuit of wealth and to paganism. The ideology that shapes Bacon's experimental program is itself a false idol.

While Bacon acknowledges the limitations of the human senses, he suggests that the use of technological instruments can compensate for these, "for no man, be he never so cunning and practiced, can make a straight line or perfect circle by steadiness of hand, which may be easily done by help of a ruler and compass."[25] Donne's critique of natural philosophy encompasses both the senses and the instruments that Bacon proposes as "ague":

> When wilt thou shake of this Pedantery,
> Of being taught by sense and Fantasy?
> Thou look'st through spectacles; small things seeme great,
> Below; But vp into the watch-towre get,
> And see all things despoyld of fallacies:
> Thou shalt not peepe through lattices of eies,
> Nor heare through Laberinths of eares, nor learne
> By circuit, or collections to discerne,
> In heauen thou straight know'st all, concerning it,
> And what concerns it not, shall straight forget. (SA 291–300)

Donne's critique of the capacity of technology to compensate for the limitations of human senses parallels the insights that Montaigne offers in *The Apology of Raymond Sebond,* in which he observes that "our condition appropriating things unto it selfe, and transforming them to its owne humour: wee know no more how things are in sooth and truth; For: *nothing comes unto us but falsified and altered by our senses.* Where the compass, the quadrant or the ruler are crooked: all proportions drawne by them, and all the buildings erected by their measure, are also necessarily defective and imperfect." It is impossible to find a standard against which our own judgments and the accuracy of our technological devices can be measured: "To judge of the apparences that we receive of subjects, we had need have a judicatorie instrument: to verifie this instrument, we should have demonstration; and to approve demonstration, an instrument: thus are we ever turning round."[26] For Donne, technological instruments that would ostensibly compensate for the limitations of the senses guarantee no more clarity than "lattices of eies." The new technology simply multiplies the distortions and weakness of the senses. The objects it studies remain discrete particulars of an imperfect knowledge that must and will be forgotten when the soul ascends to heaven.

If the poet of the *Anniversaries* pronounces that "to try truth forth is far more trouble than this world is worth," the persistent preoccupation of the poems is with demystifying the political processes that validate claims about the world and elevate them to the status of truth. The origins of Bacon's experimental strategies, as Martin has pointed out, lie in the procedures through which fact is constructed in the courtroom.[27] While matters of "fact" in the courtroom are determined through a process of information gathering, testimony, and disputation, and as such are recognized as human artifacts, Bacon confers upon his own experimental procedures the status of infallibility and political neutrality.

Donne may be seen as appropriating aspects of Bacon's critique of systematizing while nevertheless critiquing Bacon's attack on the "fictions and fantasies" of astronomers and natural philosophers who presume upon the capacity of "human actions and arts" to incarnate some image of divine order. For Donne, these "fictions and fantasies," when recognized as such—as conspicuously limited human attempts to represent the divine on earth—at their best, like his own art, nevertheless engender some measure of beauty and order that point at least in the direction of the divine. The ordered chaos of the poems is represented as the result of a specific ban that has been enacted against these attempts to enter into "commerce" with heaven:

> What Artist now dares boast that he can bring
> Heauen hither, or constellate any thing,
> So as the influence of those starres may bee
> Imprisond in an Herbe, or Charme, or Tree,
> And doe by touch, all which those starres could do?
> The art is lost, and correspondence too.
> For heauen giues little, and the earth takes lesse,
> And man least knowes their trade, and purposes.
> If this commerce 'twixt heauen and earth were not
> Embarr'd, and all this trafique quite forgot,
> Shee, for whose losse we haue lamented thus,
> Would worke more fully'and pow'rfully on vs. (FA 391–402)

Donne's reference to "trade[s] and purposes" refers both to men's ignorance of signs of God's work on earth and to men's ignorance of the responsibilities and limits that attend their social positions.[28] The passage is almost certainly a reference to Bacon's attack in *The Advancement of Learning* on the widely held belief in the correspondence between the microcosm and the macrocosm. He states that "the ancient opinion that man was Microcosmus, an abstract or model of the world, hath been fantastically strained by Paracelsus and the alchemists, as if there were to be found in man's body certain correspondences and parallels, which should have respect to all varieties of things, as stars, plants and minerals, which are extant in the great world."[29] While Donne may himself be skeptical of the claims of Paracelsus and the alchemists, he seems to find their notion of *sympathy* between humankind and the cosmos more attractive than Bacon's rhetoric of torture and mastery. For Donne, the impulse to see "correspondences and parallels" between heaven and earth underlies all artistic endeavors, which at their best are acts of worship. The real danger, Donne suggests, arises not from the "fantastically strained" claims of Paracelsus and the alchemists but from Bacon's attempts to regulate and censor such claims and to present himself as uniquely capable of locating legitimate expressions of divine will on earth.

The playful participation of the central "she" of the poems in the creation of the world provides a model in the "Second Anniversary" for human acts of creativity that are compatible with a voluntarist theology:

> When nature was most busie, the first weeke,
> Swadling the new-borne earth, God seemd to like
> That she should sport herselfe sometimes, and play,
> To mingle and vary colours euery day:
> And then, as though she could not make inow,
> Himselfe his various Rainbow did allow. (FA 347–52)

"She" is closely identified, if not conflated, with the beauty of the feminized nature in which "she" revels; this close identification undermines the strategies for control and domination over nature, which Bacon's experimental program promotes and justifies. "She" models human creation as noncoercive and respectful of the beauty and benevolence of nature.

In associating the central "she" with the beauty of the natural world, Donne preserves the necessity of God's voluntary participation in nature and resists attempts to reduce nature to an image of temporal, monarchical power.

> [S]hee, in whom all white, and redde,.and blue
> (Beautyies ingredients) voluntary grew,

As in an unuext Paradise, from whom
Did all things verdure, and their lustre come,
Whose composition was miraculous,
Being all color, all Diaphanous . . .
Shee, shee is dead; shee's dead. (FA 361–66, 369)

The lines explicitly associate color and beauty with the prelapsarian
world, implicitly rendering them signs of God's voluntary presence
in the natural world. Color and beauty are represented as essential,
rather than accidental, attributes of "she" because, while they are
evident to the "noblest sense" and provide "proof" of God's presence
in nature, they are "incorporeal," not quantifiable or subject to
control.[30] These emblems of divine omnipotence—and implicitly,
of human freedom—the poet suggests, are in danger of being
displaced by "bought colours" which "illude mens sense" and
should "more affright, then pleasure thee." The lines call the reader
to scrutinize the political motives that underlie constructions of
God in nature and gesture toward the role that the economy of
Jacobean patronage plays in legitimating claims about the divine
order in nature. Punning off the word *sense*, the lines may be read as
implicating interpretations and representations of nature that
ostensibly correct the limitations of the senses in the erosion of
individual freedom and judgment.

The passage may also offer a specific theological critique of the
concept of "natural law," in which the "miraculous" and voluntary
workings of God in nature are reduced to mere clockwork. As
Donne's lines suggest, the image of God that the natural philoso-
pher reveals is not that of an omnipotent God, whose will is
expressed freely in nature, but one whose workings are reduced to
rules of law that threaten to take precedence over his will. In the age
of precise knowledge of the laws of nature, "miracles," as Donne
conceived of them anyway, would be displaced by the technological
wonders that captured the imagination of the court elite and fed it

with dreams of imperialist power. The passage points to the dangers of conferring exclusive authority over nature to an interpretive elite that is driven by transparently political motives. In this respect, the role that court politics plays in legitimating representations of nature serves as a specific instance of a general corruption. Despite whatever aesthetic gratification the poet provides in incarnating some image in his verse of the lost "beauty" and "color" associated with the central "she," the *Anniversaries*, contra Bacon's narrow definition of poetry, are, the lines suggest, intended more to "affright" than "pleasure" the reader.

V

Insofar as "she" is identified with a merciful and loving God, "she" also provides, for Donne, an image of the ideal monarch. "She" is depicted as using her prerogative both to weed out the "pride" of corrupt courtiers and to alleviate the suffering that stems from the miscarriage of justice. At the same time, she submits her actions to her own standard of justice:

> . . . shee gaue pardons and was liberall,
> For, onely her selfe except, shee pardond all:
> Shee coynd, in this, that her impressions gaue
> To all our actions the worth they haue:
> Shee gaue protections; the thoughts of her brest
> Satans rude Officers could nere arrest.
> As these prerogatiues being met in one,
> Made her a soueraign state, religion
> Made her a Church; and these two made her all.
> Shee who was all this All, and could not fall
> To worse, by company, (for shee was still
> More Antidote, then all the world as ill)
> Shee, shee doth leaue it, and by Death, suruiue. (SA 368–79)

The proper exercise of the monarch's prerogative is implicitly compared to the divine and voluntary grace of God, whose "impressions gave / To all our actions all the worth they have." Donne's political investment in a voluntarist theology is evident in his suggestion that the promise of salvation is sufficient motivation for a moral existence and leads man to "strive / The more"; James need not impose more restrictions on man in this respect than God himself has. The emphasis Donne places on the role that the prerogative plays in tempering the justice of her courts contrasts to Bacon's reflections on the unrestrained exercise of the prerogative, in which he emphasizes that "our Sovereign hath both an enlarging and restraining liberty of her Prerogative: that is she hath power to set at liberty things restrained by statute law or otherwise" and also to "restrain things that are at liberty."³¹ Donne, who had witnessed the immediate implications for his family of the monarch's power to restrain, conspicuously omits mention of that "right." As in the preface to *Pseudo-Martyr*, he emphasizes instead the monarch's responsibility in protecting her subjects from persecution.

The introduction of "he" in line 380 subtly shifts the focus of the passage cited above; the subsequent lines address a specific individual—possibly one numbering among the "company" to whose evil influence "she" is impervious. In the lines that follow, Donne's reference to distinguishing between accidental and essential joys addresses a key hermeneutical problem within Bacon's quest for divine law in nature:

> All this, in Heauen; whither who doth not striue
> The more, because shee's there, he doth not know
> That accidentall ioyes in Heauen do grow.
> But pause, My soule, and study ere thou fall
> On accidentall ioyes, th'essentiall.
> Still before Accessories doe abide
> A triall, must the principall be tride. (SA 380–86)

Donne's lines recognize the truth that Bacon himself equivocally invokes, that one can never presume upon the congruity between human evaluations and distinctions and those made by God. To claim to know what "joys" or qualities are essential is to claim to know God, the lines suggest. Any taxonomic or experimental strategy that seeks to make these absolute distinctions is an attempt to subject God to "trial," to hold him accountable to human values and judgments. Insofar as the monarch is the human representative of divine law, such strategies, as Donne suggests in his sermon at Whitehall, must also be attempts to delimit the authority of the king. At the same time, however, the final lines are sufficiently ambiguous to suggest also that the king, along with his "accessories," may also be called to account for his actions. This reading is reinforced by the implied contrast between the ideal "she" who "could not fall / To worse by company" and the current—and possibly future—kings who allow themselves to manipulated by the status-hungry courtiers who encircle them.

Though the "she" of the *Anniversaries* can be trusted not to abuse her absolute power, Donne's qualification that she "still was more antidote than the world was ill" reflects his resistance to any political "physic" that might involve the enlargement of the king's prerogative. In the fallen world of the *Anniversaries*, the absence of the ideal monarch becomes a model for government on earth. The passage, which seems to echo Bacon's reflections on the learnedness of Salomon, follows, significantly, upon Donne's dismissal of the technological accuracy promised by the New Philosophy and his analogy between the limitations of the circuit court and the collection of data:

> There thou (but in no other schoole) maist bee
> Perchance, as learned, and as full, as shee,
> Shee who all libraries had throughly red
> At home in her owne thoughts, and Practised

So much good as would make many more:
Shee whose example they must all implore,
Who would or doe, or thinke well, and confesse
That aie the vertuous Actions they expresse
Are but a new, and worse edition
Of her some one thought, or one action:
Shee, who in th'Art of knowing Heauen, was growen
Here vpon Earth, to such perfection,
That shee hath, euer since to Heauen shee came,
(In a far fairer print), but read the same:
Shee, shee not satisfied with all this waite,
(For so much knowledge, as would ouer-fraite
Another, did but Ballast her) is gone
As well t'enioy, as get perfectione.
And cals vs after her, in that shee tooke,
(Taking herselfe) our best, and worthiest booke. (SA 301–20)

The only monarch who can justly lay claim to exercise perfect justice
and to embody the divine power and knowledge of God is Donne's
feminized embodiment of God. Because she functions as the ideal
reader and text of the Books of Nature and Scripture, her absence
from the earth makes definitive readings of both impossible. The
temporal monarch, James—and Henry in his turn—can hope only
to approximate divine truth, virtue, and justice by acknowledging
that their knowledge and power are limited in relationship to hers,
that the most "virtuous actions" that they can "express / Are but a
new and worse edition / Of her some one thought, or one action."
In characterizing her as "our best and worthiest book," moreover,
"she" becomes that which resists interpretation. In this respect, her
textualization makes her the embodiment of the spirit, rather than
the letter of the law. While divine knowledge is the "ballast" of
God, the claim to divine knowledge, the poet warns, can only "over-
freight" the mortal king—and in turn, breed civil unrest.

VI

The poems, finally, provide important sight into Donne's refusal
in 1611 and 1612 to take holy orders, as they demonstrate the poet's
ambivalence, if not resistance, to the compromises demanded by the
entire economy of patronage and power in which the church is also
fully implicated:

> Returne not, my soul, from this extasee,
> And meditation of what thou shalt be,
> To earthly thoughts, till it thee appeare,
> With whom thy conuersation must be there.
> With whom wilt thou Conuerse? what station
> Canst thou chose out, free from infection,
> That wil not giue thee theirs, nor drink in thine?
> Shalt thou not find a spungy slack Diuine
> Drink and Sucke in th'Instructions of Great men,
> And for the word of God, vent them again?
> Are there not some Courts (And then, no things bee
> So like as Courts) which, in this let vs see,
> That wits and tongues of Libellars are weak
> Because they do more ill, than these can speake?
> The poyson' is gone through all, poysons affect
> Chiefly the cheefest parts, but some effect
> In Nailes, and Haires, yea excrements, will show;
> So will poyson of sinne, in the most low.
> Vp, vp, my drowsie soul, where thy new eare
> Shall in the Angels songs no discord heare. . . . (SA 321–40)

For Donne, at least in 1611 and 1612, to take holy orders is to take
the orders of the monarch. From the "spongy slack divine" to the
highest of courtiers, all are implicated for Donne in drinking and
sucking the word of great men and venting it out out again as the

word of God. The question beginning in line 331 is deliberately—and characteristically—ambiguous. The lines can be read as an attack on the "wits and tongues of libellers" who may yet be incapable of effacing the good performed within the court, or as a suggestion that the "wits and tongues of libellers are weak" because their accusations cannot possibly match the degree of illness that pervades the court. The former reading provides, of course, some slight defense against the charge of libel that the poems may themselves engender. However, the lines are a damning critique of both the courts of law and the court of James. Donne's experience within these overlapping spheres of political power leads him to believe that judge, courtier, and even king, are more corrupt than those individuals at the bottom of the social hierarchy who are subject to their power and judgment. Those who hold the greatest power, Donne suggests, have the least credibility to lay claim to divine justice and truth.

For Donne, the "angel's song" is audible only to those who distinguish between divine truth and human constructions, and who acknowledge the extent to which all the artifacts constructed within the economy of patronage and court—the decisions that pass for justice in the courts, the interpretations that are rendered of the Books of Nature and Scripture—are, like his poems, shaped to some extent by its corrupt demands. For Donne, whose exile had taught him the tenuousness of courtly power and influence, Bacon is representative of the failure of so many courtiers to recognize that their social identities, like Bacon's interpretations of nature and law, are themselves accidental rather than essential, mere frippery that, like the sails in "The Calm," can be torn to shreds by a strong wind. Bacon's growing confidence in his position and influence is as misguided as his confidence in his attempts to confine God to the certainty of natural law:

> But could this low world ioyes essentiall touch,
> Heauens accidentall ioyes would passe them much.

> How poore and lame, must then our casuall bee?
> If thy Prince will his subiects to call thee
> My Lord, and this doe swell thee, thou art than,
> By being a greater, growen to be lesse Man.
> When no Physician of redresse can speake,
> A ioyfull casuall violence may breake
> A dangerous Apostem in thy brest;
> And whilst thou ioyest in this, the dangerous rest,
> The bag may rise vp and so strangle thee.
> What eie was casuall, may euer bee.
> What should the Nature change? or make the same
> Certaine, which was but casuall, when it came?
> All casuall ioye doth loud and plainly say,
> Onely by comming that it can away.
> Onely in Heauen ioies strength is neuer spent;
> And accidentall things are permanent. (SA 471–98)

Bacon's arrogant claim to be able to distinguish between essential and accidental qualities becomes an image of the inability—which Donne remarks upon in his sermon at Whitehall—to distinguish between the arguably fortunate "accidents" that have propelled him to power and the essential will of God and sovereign, between the accidental satisfactions of earthly and courtly existence and the essential joys of heaven. The voluntary workings of God and nature serve, Donne suggests, as a reminder of the instability of temporal power and privilege.

In the lines that immediately follow on the passage above, Donne suggests that divine agency alone is capable of restoring natural order and implicitly contrasts the endless improvements in nature to be effected by divine agency to the empty and arrogant promises of the natural philosopher whose imminent political fall Donne predicts:

> Ioy of that last great Consummation
> Approches in the resurrection;

> When earthly bodies more celestiall
> Shalbe, then Angels were, for they could fall;
> This kind of ioy doth euery day admit
> Degrees of grouth, but none of loosing it.
> In this fresh ioy, tis no small part, that shee,
> Shee, in whose goodnesse, he that names degree,
> Doth iniure her; (Tis losse to be cald best,
> There where the stuffe is not such as the rest)
> Shee, who left such a body, as euen shee
> Onely in Heauen could learne, how it can bee
> Made better. (SA 491–503)

The "Physician of Redresse" may be God or the poet himself, whose voice is one of the many that are marginalized and silenced in the face of tyrannical claims to absolute truth, while the treacherous elements suggested by the phrase "the dangerous rest" may. "rise up and so strangle" both king and courtier/counselor. The "dangerous rest" may also refer, however, to hermeneutic strategies that would enshrine and enforce claims to divine truth rather than fostering an ongoing dialogue and meditation upon the nature of truth and justice. Bacon's attempt to preserve the "degree" of the king's power by defining it—as Martin suggests—through his strategies for the reform of the common law and natural philosophy, and his struggle to define his own privileged position at court in the process, breed only divisiveness and chaos. The desire of both king and courtier "to be cald best," to be considered different "stuffe" from "the rest" (499–500), creates opposition and illness in the body politic.

In contrast to the divisiveness of natural philosophy and astronomy, Donne's "she" is the subtle knot that knits together the fraying strands of court and country. As a metaphor for metaphor, "she" demonstrates the irreducibly dialogical nature of all representation, the contingency of all truth claims, and the capacity of metaphor to reconcile multiple and conflicting claims and meanings. At the same time, however, Donne's equivocal "she" embodies the confusion of degree that is the result of courtly flattery, of the willingness of courtiers—encouraged by the highest patron in the land—to deify their patrons, and themselves in the process. Though the poems specifically target natural philosophy and astronomy for the new roles that they threaten to play in legitimating James's absolutist claims, the *Anniversaries* also implicate poetry in their encompassing critique of the ideological and material interests that shape representation within the Jacobean court. If the poet prominently foregrounds the contingency of his own poetic claims, that acknowledgment, it must be noted, is itself mobilized to advance the poet's albeit ironic argument for his own advancement within the Jacobean patronage economy. In this sense, the poems provide an argument for scrutinizing the variable uses of the rhetoric of contingency. The rhetoric of contingency, as I explore more fully in the next two chapters, figures prominently among the literary technologies used to legitimate the experimental findings and theoretical claims of the Royal Society in the latter half of the seventeenth century.

3

THE FALL OF SCIENCE IN BOOK 8 OF PARADISE LOST

In the years following his death, Bacon's role as a defender of monarchical absolutism was effaced, and his name and rhetoric were increasingly invoked to legitimate theories and practices that reflected a broad spectrum of political opinions, including those of moderate and radical Puritans who believed that progressive knowledge of nature and the body—and of the applied sciences of husbandry and medicine, in particular—would play a central role in bringing about some version of a Puritan millenium.[1] The Third Prolusion, an attack on scholastic philosophy written at the close of Milton's studies at Cambridge, testifies to the poet's early enthusiasm for natural philosophy, as he reflects on a coming flowering of knowledge of the natural world: "How much more satisfaction there would be, gentlemen, and how much worthier it would be of your name to rove with your eyes over all the lands which are drawn on the map . . . [and] then to search out and examine the natures of all living creatures; and from them to turn to the study of all living creatures; and from them to turn to the study of the hidden virtues of stones and herbs."[2] In the promethean dreams of the youthful poet, the most "hidden virtues" of nature are made evident to man, mobilized in the service of Puritan gentlemen, whose pious and all-knowing gaze—and administration—encompasses all of creation. Milton likely shared the conviction of Puritan reformers, including those of the Hartlib circle, with whom he had significant contact in the 1640s, that medicine and natural philosophy, in particular the applied science of husbandry, would serve as instruments to ameliorate the moral and material conditions of the citizens of the English Commonwealth.[3]

By the early 1660s, however, Milton had ample reason to suspect that under the auspices of the Royal Society, natural philosophy heralded not the creation of the Puritan "New Jerusalem" on earth but a church-dominated state antithetical to Milton's own belief in the priesthood of all believers, and an aggressive capitalism that would expand the geographical reach of the restored monarchy. Book 8 of *Paradise Lost* provides strong indications that the natural philosophy that a youthful Milton appears to have embraced as an instrument in the realization of the Puritan millenium was, for the aging defender of a dead Commonwealth, identified with the abandonment of republican ideals for political and economic self-interest, with the abstractions of the academy, and with the authoritative claims of the monarchy and established clergy against the interpretive freedom of the spiritually enlightened individual.[4] The dialogue on astronomy, moreover, demonstrates the poet's complex awareness of the role that patriarchal ideology plays in buttressing the authority of the monarch and the landed elite and the privilege they claim to exploit and exhaust the natural resources upon which the entire nation depended.

I

The controversy between John Wilkins and Alexander Ross over the relationship between natural philosophy and astronomy, on the one hand, and Scripture, on the other, provides important insights into the specific nature of the concerns that the poet raises in the dialogue on astronomy in book 8. Wilkins's *The Discovery of a World, or A Discourse Tending to Prove That 'Tis Probable There May Be Another Habitable World in That Planet* (1638) and *Discourse Concerning a New Planet* (1640), together with Alexander Ross's vituperative critique of Wilkins's claims entitled *The New Planet No Planet, or The Earth No Wandering Star Except in the Wandring Heads of Galileans* (1646), as Grant McColley first observed in 1937, provide the principal source materials for the dialogue between Adam and Raphael.[5] Alastair Fowler has challenged McColley's original claim that Wilkins's and Ross's writings served, respectively, as the source for Adam's and Raphael's parts in the dialogue, noting that Wilkins's writings inform the parts of both Raphael and Adam.[6] The question remains, however, why the poet, who appears to pay tribute in book 5 to Galileo as the "Tuscan artist" (288), would in book 8 fashion an angelic representative whose responses to Adam's astronomical speculations so closely resemble the observations of a vocal critic of natural philosophy and astronomy—and one whom Nicolson has dubbed a "crusted conservative."[7] As a champion of free expression, of revolution and regicide, Milton lay at the opposite end of the political and theological spectrum from Ross. Appropriating elements of the conservative critique of astronomy and natural philosophy may, however, have allowed Milton to accomplish the dual purposes of circumventing the censorship of the restored monarchy and pitting one defender of the status quo against another to further his own ends. A precedent for this tactic can be found in the radical Henry Stubbe, who, as J. R. Jacob argues, consistently adopted and adapted conservative positions in order to undermine conservative ideologies.[8]

During the Restoration, leading figures in the Royal Society, including Wilkins and Boyle, represented natural philosophy as fulfilling an important theological and ideological function in England, in demonstrating the divine, and unquestionably hierarchical, order imprinted in the Book of Nature. Boyle was a likely source for Milton's knowledge of the activities of the Royal Society; Milton was tutor to the sons of Boyle's sister, Lady Ranelagh, and it was through the intervention of Boyle and Ranelagh that Milton escaped execution at the Restoration. Boyle and Wilkins represented natural philosophy as an antidote to both Hobbesian materialism and the threat posed by sectarian enthusiasts, who invoked Scripture to support radical challenges to the monarch and the privileges of the landed elite. Natural philosophy, under the aegis of the Royal Society, could therefore buttress Anglican theology against radical readings of both the Book of Scripture and the Book of Nature by providing a conservative and unassailable reading of God's design in nature. The establishment of the Royal Society promised to make the interpretation of the Book of Nature a skill accessible only to those male members of the upper classes who endorsed and were endorsed by the Royal Society. Under the auspices of the Royal Society, then, natural philosophy would realize some semblance of Bacon's vision by displacing the individual interpretation of Scripture, associated with the political corruptions of the imagination and the political disorder and chaos of the 1640s, with a consensual, authoritative determination of meaning.

At least theoretically, most members of the Royal Society insisted upon the auxiliary and subordinate relationship of the book of nature to that of Scripture, and upon the individual's freedom to interpret scripture. Boyle's *The Excellency of Theology, as Compar'd with Natural Philosophy* (1674) self-consciously posits the inadequacy of natural philosophy to provide complete and definitive knowledge of God. The Book of Nature was, Boyle suggests, structured like a romance in which the "parts have such a connection and relation to one another, and the things we would discover are so darkly and incompleatly knowable by those that precede them, that the mind is never satisfied till it comes to the end of the Book."[9] The "end," or the totally comprehensive theory, was for Boyle endlessly deferred to revelation, and the emphasis placed instead on the utility of individual "facts." The creation of philosophical systems, Boyle warned, would ultimately contribute to an understanding of the Book of Nature as conceptually independent from and equal, if not superior, to Scripture. "It has long seem'd to me," writes Boyle in

Certain Physiological Essays (1661) "none of the least impediments of the real advancement of true natural philosophy that men have been so *forward to write systems*."[10] However, as Markley has argued, for Boyle and other members of the Royal Society, the analogical relationship of nature to Scripture confers semiotic coherence upon the Book of Nature, thereby authorizing the evidence of divine order that the natural philosopher locates in nature.[11] At the same time, this analogical relationship alternately justifies the attempts of the pious natural philosopher to refashion technologically and conceptually a fallen and chaotic natural world into an idealized image of divine order.

The high church Anglican Alexander Ross was among the most vocal critics of the Royal Society; since the early 1640s he had charged that, far from reinforcing theological orthodoxy, the claims of natural philosophers and astronomers undermined the authority of scripture and threatened the power of the clergy. If Milton's Raphael may indeed, as McColley argued, ventriloquize Ross, the poet would certainly have had altogether different reasons for insisting on the primacy of scripture over that of natural philosophy and astronomy. Milton's persistent belief in the individual's right to interpret Scripture is evident in his attack on the clergy in *A Readie and Easie Way* (1660), in which he suggests that clerical authority is antithetical to both "Spiritual or Civil Liberty" in which "the whole freedom of Man consists":

Who can enjoy any thing in this World with contentment, who hath not liberty to serve God, and to save his own Soul, according to the best Light which God hath planted in him to that purpose, by the reading of his reveal'd Will, and the guidance of his Holy Spirit? That this is best pleasing to God, and that the whole Protestant Church allows no supream Judg or Rule in Matters of Religion, but the Scriptures; and these to be interpreted by the Scriptures themselves, which necessarily infers Liberty of Conscience.[12]

If Ross perceived astronomy as a threat to the authority of Scripture and clergy, Milton is more likely to have lumped the astronomer together with the cleric and seen both as threatening the "Liberty of Conscience" of the individual whose access to divine truth lay in Scripture alone.

A brief consideration of Wilkins's career will serve to illuminate some of the complex reasons that may have shaped Milton's choice of Wilkins' writings on astronomy as the principle target of what I will argue is a broader ideological critique of the activities of the Royal Society in book 8. Wilkins was one of the most active and prominent members of the Society. He played a key role in its formation in helping to draft—and some years later, redraft—the charter; together with Henry Oldenburg, he served as secretary to the newly formed organization, and in 1663 went on to become vice-president, and to serve for years on its policy-making council.[13] The most visible proponent of the Copernican worldview in England, Wilkins took a leading role in the Society in advocating the pursuit of astronomical studies. Before the Civil War *The Discovery of a World in the Moone* enjoyed a great deal of popularity. The basis for Fontanelle's extremely popular *Conversations on the Plurality of Worlds*, Wilkins's treatment of "lunar inhabitants and interplanetary travel" was, as Shapiro has noted, the "chief source of the wider literary currency given these ideas" in the late seventeenth and early eighteenth centuries.[14]

Long before the Restoration, when he would assume high-ranking positions in both the Anglican Church and the Royal Society, Wilkins had made a career of siding with institutional authority against the interests of the radical Puritan reformers. Though himself a Puritan, and brother-in-law to Cromwell, Wilkins nevertheless maintained a reputation as a protector of known royalists during the Interregnum—which earned him an easy and prompt transition into public office under the restored monarchy. Wilkins shared the belief with other members of the Royal Society, and with Bacon before them, that natural philosophy would uncover the "real" order of nature and in turn provide an unquestionable foundation for the government of men. In *A Discourse Concerning the Beauty of Providence* (1649), Wilkins represents natural theology—that is, theology based in arguments from both reason and natural order—as an antidote to the threat posed by radical interpretations of events in the natural and political worlds, two realms that he frequently conflates throughout the work. "It cannot but occasion some suggestions of Diffidence and Infidelitie," observes Wilkins, "to consider those many strange revolutions and changes in the world, which in outward appearance, seem so full of disorder and wilde contingencies." Wilkins goes on to suggest that the "oppression" that his fellow countrymen confront seems likely to drive even "a wise man" to the brink of madness: "that is, puts him to his wits end, transports him with wilde imaginations."¹⁵ Wilkins soothes the anxious reader who is confronted with a world turned upside down. Natural theology, he suggests, provides assurance of the divine, hierarchical order in nature that will in time prevail against the madness of radical sectarian enthusiasts.

Throughout his career, Wilkins consistently maintains belief in a divinely sanctioned hierarchical order. His resistance to the revolutionary upheaval of the traditional hierarchies in English culture is evident in his project of demonstrating the order that underlies apparent chaos. Invoking Ecclesiastes 10:7, he consoles the reader who confronts what appears to be the "total subversion of those degrees, in which the order and harmony of things doth consist, *Servants being on horses, and Princes walking as servants on the earth: When the mountains are removed, and the pillars of the earth tremble.* When Religion and Laws (which are the foundations of a people) are out of course." Far from fomenting this revolutionary inversion of the natural order, Wilkins offers his readers a dose of rhetorical Prozac, counseling them that

What ever comes to passe shall be *beautiful,* and therefore should be *welcome.* All things that befall us, shal lead us on to the same journey's end, Happiness. And therefore we should not in our expectation of future matters ingage our selves in the desire of any particular successe; but with a *travailer's* indifferency (as *Epictetus* speaks in *Arian*) who when he comes to doubtful turnings, doth not desire one way should be more true than another. So should we entertain every thing that we meet with in our passage through this life Especially since we are sure, that there is none of them, but (if we belong to God) shall further in us that which is our main businesse, our *journey* to happinesse.[16]

If one falls victim to hunger, injustice, or injury on one's journey to Happiness, it ought not undermine one's faith in the divinely decreed natural order of things, particularly since it is frequently the case that "his own sin and neglect hath occasioned them."[17] Shapiro notes that the "doctrine of Providence" that Wilkins advances in this work "provided a rationalization for the political inaction and passive adaptation to political change that Wilkins himself practiced." Far from preaching revolution, Wilkins counsels the reader to acquiesce to the status quo, and to defer judgment before those with privileged insight into the *"works of Creation,"* and into the "rank and station" of each element of creation in the divinely decreed hierarchy.[18] For Wilkins, social station and wealth provide confirmation of moral standing.

In light of her observations on *A Discourse Concerning the Beauty of Providence*, Shapiro's characterization of Wilkins in her biographical study published in 1969 seems at once humorous and disturbing. Wilkins, she observes, "was no rebel, but a man squarely within the main intellectual currents of his time. In short, Wilkins was a moderate, the kind of person whom we have all encountered, whom none of us find strange, and indeed with whom most of us identify." Shapiro's description serves well to demonstrate why Milton would have viewed Wilkins with both suspicion and disdain. While, as Shapiro observes, Wilkins was "lauded by his friends," ostensibly for the "political astuteness with which he pursued his own essentially moral goals through the political maze," he was "attacked by his enemies for unprincipled cultivation of whoever held power at the moment." In 1660, shortly after the publication of *A Ready and Easy Way*, intended to forestall the return of the monarchy, with Milton still at risk for defending regicide, Wilkins, brother-in-law to Cromwell, received a royal appointment as dean of Ripon.[19] On November 28 of that year, Wilkins presided over the meeting that resulted in the decision to petition the monarch for the foundation of the Royal Society.

Milton would surely have noticed that the strategy Wilkins used to reconcile Copernicanism with the authority of Scripture is identical to his strategy for addressing the threat posed by radical interpretations of Scripture. Wilkins's approach is simple enough: Biblical passages that support his theories about lunar inhabitants are to be taken literally. Passages that contradict his claims are merely metaphorical, using "vulgar expressions" to render them accessible to the unenlightened rabble, who are nevertheless incapable of discerning the underlying the meaning of Scripture—or divine order in the cosmos—without the guiding hand of Wilkins himself. Discussing biblical passages that contradict his claims, he asserts that

the phrases which the Holy Ghost uses concerning these things are not to be understood in a literall sense; but rather as vulgar expressions, and this rule is set downe by Saint *Austin*, where speaking concerning that in the Psalme, *who stretched the earth upon the waters*, hee notes, that when the words of Scripture shall seeme to contradict common sense or experience, there are they to be understood in a qualified sense, and not according to the letter. And 'tis observed that for want of this rule, some of the ancients have fastened strange absurdities upon the words of the Scripture. So Saint *Ambrose* esteemed it a heresie, to thinke, that the Sunne and starres were not very hot, as being against the words of Scripture. . . . These and such like absurdities have followed, when men looke for the grounds of Philosophie in the words of Scripture.

Wilkins himself, however, frequently looks to ground philosophy in Scripture, using it to legitimate his cosmological speculations. He finds support in Scripture, for example, for his assertion that the moon's "Orbe is not solid" and that in fact all the planetary orbs are "all of a fluid (perhaps aereous) substance."[20] Wilkins follows a parallel strategy in his use of patristic and classical sources, invoking Augustine, *Sixtus Senensis*'s biblical annotations, and a host of other classical and early Christian sources to support the same claim. Insofar as he draws upon whatever arguments are at hand, Wilkins's strategies for verifying his claims challenge Whiggish accounts of the "rise of science" and demonstrate that the line between the ancients and the moderns in the period is indeed a shifting one. As an antidote to the anarchy of individual interpretations spawned by the doctrine of the "inner light," Wilkins's "method" for selectively interpreting metaphor legitimates the authority of an interpretive elite whose shared ideology marks them as qualified readers.

Wilkins's attack on Hobbes's attempts to provide a foundation for a stable social order in a system based on "infallible and mathematical certainty" rather than Scripture may be seen, in this regard, as an attempt to deflect attention from the problematic relationship between Scripture and his own arguments from natural theology. In the posthumously published *Principles and Duties of Natural Religion* (1675) Wilkins implicitly attacks Hobbes for undermining the authority of Scripture: "If we suppose God to have made any Revelation of his Will to mankind, can any man propose or fancy any better way for conveying down to Posterity the Certainty of it, than that clear and universal Tradition which we have for the History of the Gospel? And must not that man be very unreasonable, who will not be content with as much evidence for an *ancient Book* or *matter of Fact*, as any thing of that nature is capable of?"[21] Wilkins rewrites history to erase the role that competing interpretations of Scripture played in fomenting a bloody Civil War; his belief in a "clear and universal Tradition" self-evident in

Scripture can be sustained only by limiting interpretation to a highly select readership and by effectively marginalizing competing interpretations as vulgar or politically motivated misprisions. Wilkins's statements affirming the centrality of Scripture frequently seem little more than perfunctory gestures that do little to mask the nearly autonomous status he assigns astronomy and natural philosophy.

Despite Wilkins's claims that astronomy and natural philosophy will buttress belief and implicitly marginalize radical readings of the Books of Nature and Scripture, Ross attacks Wilkins for undermining the authoritative status of Scripture: "Take heed you play not the Anatomist upon these celestiall bodies, (whose inward parts are hid from you) in the curious and needlesse search of them; you may well lose your selfe, but this way you shall never finde God. . . . Whereas you say, That *Astronomy serves to confirme the truth of the holy Scripture:* you are very preposterous, for you will not have the truth of Scripture affirmed by Astronomie, but you will have the truth of Astronomie confirmed by Scripture."[22] In effect, Ross argues that Wilkins's principal concern is in securing knowledge of the heavens, rather than of God. For Wilkins, astronomical "truths" are the primary texts for which Scripture provides secondary confirmation. Ross warns Wilkins that theories of cosmic order are subject to endless contestation and revision and are, in this respect, a much more precarious ground than Scripture upon which to build belief. If Wilkins believes that astronomy and natural theology, in unveiling the hierarchical creative order of God, will provide an effective weapon against radical challenges to the status quo, Ross astutely anticipates that these discourses will ultimately displace scriptural authority and—perhaps more importantly for Ross—the traditional authority of the clergy.

The anticlerical Milton appropriates elements of Ross's critique to undermine attempts by Wilkins and other members of the Royal Society to employ natural philosophy as a corrective to skepticism and, more importantly, to radical interpretations of Scripture. If

Milton concedes with Raphael that "heaven / Is as the book of God before thee set" (66–67), the dialogue on astronomy severely circumscribes the kinds of knowledge one reads in the heavens and suggests that the motives one brings to the reading are crucial.[23] "Ask[ing] and search[ing]" (66) are not in themselves blameworthy when the questions are finally referred to Raphael, the "divine / Historian" (6–7) identified with Scripture, for resolution. The discussion stems from a "doubt" that Adam presents to Raphael: "Something yet of doubt remains, / Which only thy solution can resolve" (13–14). However, Milton's repeated references to Adam's "doubt" in lines 116 and 179 frame his questioning as a kind of skepticism. The emergence of astronomy, which Raphael foretells, then, is associated with the erosion of confidence in scriptural authority and the displacement of divine truth with human constructions of natural order which are conspicuously fallible."[24] In book 8, Milton, like Donne, represents astronomy as an enterprise motivated by lack of faith in a divine order and suggests that the identification of a particular model of the heavens ultimately intensifies rather than allays skepticism.

Milton emphasizes the primacy of revelation over natural philosophy in Adam's creation narrative in the second half of book 8. Creation reinforces Adam's impulse to worship; however, nature is mute in the face of his queries:

> Tell, if ye saw, how came I thus, how here?
> Not of myself; by some great Maker then?
> In goodness and in power preeminent;
> Tell me, how may I know him, how adore,
> From whom I have that thus I move and live,
> And feel that I am happier than I know. (277–82)

From his experience of his own body and of nature, Adam concludes that he did not create himself and that God is both good and all powerful; but beyond that, Adam receives from nature no answers and begins to "stray" until God voluntarily reveals himself to Adam in a dream. Significantly, when God does "endue" Adam with "sudden apprehension" of nature, the knowledge he finds in it is specific to the nature of creation. Man's moral responsibility to both God and nature, to "Till and keep" (320) the garden and refrain from eating of the "Tree whose operation brings / Knowledge of good and ill" (323–24), God states specifically. He does not leave it to Adam to "read" this crucial information from or into nature.

II

While Wilkins frames many of his astronomical claims within the rhetoric of contingency and probability, this rhetoric contrasts rather markedly to both the totalizing nature of his claims and the imperialist ideology they advance. One of the key goals of this ostensibly speculative treatise is to "prove" that the moon is in fact inhabited. Alternately invoking ostensibly empirical proof, the authority of other astronomers, Diodorus, Anaxagorus, Democritus, and Augustinus Nisus, Wilkins asserts with great assurance that the "body" of the moon is furnished with seas, rivers, mountains, valleys, and "spacious plaines," in short with the "same conveniences of habitation as this hath." Having established the point, Wilkins is ready to present as all but self-evident his assertion that the moon is in fact inhabited, "for why else did Providence furnish that place with all such conveniences of habitation as have been above declared?"[25] The contingent claims with which Wilkins began are retroactively transformed, legitimated as objective and incontrovertible facts that he uses to elicit his readers' support for his dream of exploring and, as he strongly implies, colonizing the moon.

The imperialist ambitions that fuel Wilkins's theoretical excursions into space is evident in *The Discovery of a World in the Moone*. Invoking Aristotle's skepticism regarding extraterrestrial life, Wilkins speculates that it was politically motivated:

Perhaps it was because hee feared to displease his scholler *Alexander*, of whom 'tis related that he wept to heare a disputation of another world, since he had not then attained the Monarchy of this, his restlesse wide heart would have esteemed this Globe of Earth not big enough for him, if there had beene another, which made the Satyrist say of him . . . "That he did vexe himselfe and sweate in his desires, as being pend up in a narrow roome, when hee was confin'd but to one world." Before he thought to seate himselfe next the Gods, but now when hee had done his best, hee must be content with some equall, or perhaps superiour Kings. . . . *Aristotle* himselfe was as loth to hold the possibility of a world which he could not discover, as *Alexander* was to heare of one which he could not conquer.

Wilkins, in fact, invites the reader to entertain the possibility that technological advances will render possible the colonization of the heavens, a feat of which Alexander himself could have only dreamt. Wilkins's reflections on the terrain of the moon implicitly address both the tactical problems of conquering its inhabitants and the future uses of a landscape fortified with "natures bulwarkes cast up at God Almighties owne charges." Evoking the Edenic dreams that fueled overseas exploration in the period, Wilkins entertains speculation that "Paradise was in a high elevated place, which some have conceived could bee no where but in the Moone."[26] While ostensibly eschewing any conclusive word on the matter, Wilkins confines his brief discussion of the issue to refuting objections to Eden's placement on the moon. Holding out the hope that a space program may provide the means for reclaiming Paradise, Wilkins goes on to inaugurate, at least imaginatively, the race for space.

Wilkins deploys the masculinist rhetoric of conquest that drove colonialist expansion to fuel his compatriots' dreams of inter-planetary conquest:

In the first ages of the world the Islanders either thought themselves to be the onely dwellers upon the earth, or else if there were any other, yet they could not possibly conceive how they might have any commerce with them, being severed by the deepe and broad Sea, but the after-times found out the invention of ships, in which notwithstanding none but some bold daring men durst venture, there being few so resolute as to commit themselves unto the vaste Ocean, and yet now how easie a thing is this, even to a timorous & cowardly nature? So, perhaps, there may be some other meanes invented for a conveyance to the Moone, and though it may seeme a terrible and impossible thing ever to passe through the vaste spaces of the aire, yet no question there would bee some men who durst venture this as well as the other.

In the interest of investing nationalist pride in space travel, Wilkins casts doubt upon the virility of Englishmen, suggesting that the continued failure of England to develop a conveyance for navigating space will mark them as a "timorous and cowardly" nation. He then proceeds to invoke the specter of the German conquest of the moon, noting that "*Keplar* doubts not, but that as soone as the art of flying is found out, some of their Nation will make one of the first colonies that shall inhabite that other world." His summary dismissal of this disturbing possibility—"But I leave this and the like conjectures to the fancie of the reader"—tempts his reader, seducing him with dreams of assailing vast spaces unattempted yet by men, and frightening him with nightmares of national impotency unmasked if he doesn't.[27]

The will to power that fuels Wilkins's dreams of interplanetary conquest in the late 1630s is also evident in his language projection scheme, which though already the subject of debate and discussion in the 1640s would not be published until 1668, when it appeared as *An Essay toward a Real Character and a Philosophical Language.* As Robert Stillman has observed, Wilkins's universal language scheme is intended to advance England's economic and political power; by creating a "set of universal symbols coincident with the universals of philosophical knowledge, the language would strive to enable in a more perfect commerce of symbols a more perfect commerce of things." As an antidote to a human language whose dialogical nature is a mark of fallenness, and which is therefore subject to the "monsters" of metaphor, to multiple and conflicting interpretations, and to the vagaries of "custom"—in short, to the claims of the vulgar and unruly masses—Wilkins attempts to construct an unambiguous system of representation rooted in an understanding of the true nature of things in the world. The "common assent" that Wilkins invokes in the *Real Character*, as in his earlier writings on astronomy, to legitimate his persistent belief in the hierarchical order of creation "lend[s] the appearance of eternality and universality to what are demonstrably the contingent values of a Restoration elite."[28]

Astronomy, as I have suggested, is associated in Milton's dialogue with the erosion of confidence in scriptural authority and the displacement of divine truth with human constructions of divine order that are conspicuously fallible. If Adam ostensibly sets out in a posture of reverence and humility, he is progressively seduced by his own speculations, which become, in fact, progressively less speculative. Adam's rhetoric reflects an initial acknowledgment of the contingency of sensory knowledge; he observes that the stars "*seem to roll / spaces incomprehensible*" (19–20). In his amendment to this statement, "for such / Their distance *argues*" (20–21), Adam moves from the realm of empirical, probabilistic knowledge to that of logical certainty. He projects his argument into the heavens, conflating his logic with God's, thereby limiting God to one appropriate representation of order. Adam has already fallen a bit and, moreover, introduced "disproportion" into nature. His specific reference to earth as "an atom" reduces nature and divine mystery to mechanism, to inert matter in motion. Unwittingly punning on his own name, Adam conjures for a moment the specter of man subject to the logic of *Leviathan*, pawn of an absolute monarch. The angel's subsequent statement that he is willing hypothetically to "Admi[t] motion in the heavens to show / Invalid that which thee to doubt it moved" (115–16) provides a clue to the nature of Adam's transgression. Lewalski has observed that Adam "implies the ineptitude of God in designing an apparently irrational Ptolemaic universe," but he might also be seen as presuming here that God either would not—or, perhaps worse, could not—move the heavens about the earth, thus challenging the omnipotence of God.[29]

In book 8 Adam's astronomical speculations are cast as a brand of celestial power-mongering. The "heaven" which is "buil[t] and unbuil[t]" (81) suggests the perversion by astronomy and, implicitly, also natural philosophy of a social ideal decreed by God in Scripture. By contrast, the motives that impel Eve's departure from the scene at the beginning of the dialogue, her desire to nurture the flowers that "at her coming sprung / And touched by her fair tendance gladlier grew" (46–47) suggest an ideological and epistemological alternative to Adam's astronomical speculations. In contrast to Adam's speculative astronomy, which is rooted in desire for power over Eve, and implicitly over the garden, and is implicitly associated with colonialist ambition and an unexamined belief in the privileges of a monarch and of a patriarchal elite, Eve demonstrates a firm commitment to service and, as Diane McColley has noted, to the material needs of the garden.[30] Knowledge for Eve is not something to be "acquired," nor is it an instrument through which to exert control; rather, it is the offspring of an act of love, of reverence for and recognition of the natural world. Michael Schoenfeldt has argued that Eve has a central role in Milton's epic in inaugurating the "significant forms of pre- and postlapsarian social life."[31] Insofar as knowledge for Eve takes the form of embodied practice, rather than a theoretical or speculative knowledge, she may be seen in the beginning of book 8 as modeling Milton's epistemological ideal.

The pleasure Eve anticipates in taking knowledge from her husband's lips, "from [which] / Not words alone pleased her" (56–57) may be seen as a positive alternative to Adam's abstract systematizing and, one might argue, to the language projection schemes that preoccupied Bacon, Wilkins, Comenius, and others in the seventeenth century.[32] The poet's invocation in book 7 draws a direct correlation between the "diurnal sphere" as the appropriate domain of mankind and the limitations of human language, the poet's determinedly "mortal voice." The poet's invocation of the muse serves as a reminder that even his mortal song must be assisted by the "muse," which is identified in *Paradise Lost* with a voluntaristic grace. While God is the "Author" or first creator, nature is continually reinscribed by human consciousness, even in the postlapsarian world. As Eve leads Adam to the "nuptial bower" in book 8,

> the Earth
> Gave sign of gratulation, and each Hill;
> Joyous the Birds; fresh Gales and gentle Airs
> Whisper'd it to the Woods, and from thir wings
> Flung Rose, flung Odors from the spicy Shrub,
> Disporting, till the amorous Bird of Night
> Sung Spousal. (513–19)

Adam reads into nature his own emotional and moral states, which are, however, dependent on his relationship to God. His prelapsarian articulations extend, with God's voluntarily proferred grace, the process of creation. Prelapsarian language and prelapsarian nature are therefore inextricably linked. Postlapsarian nature and language are, similarly, both functions of man's fallen moral state; their redemption can never be brought about under the auspices of a political structure that Milton associates with the Antichrist. Their redemption awaits the final voluntary intercession of God on earth with the coming of the millenium. And in the meantime, there's the pleasure of metaphor. For Milton, humans participate through the play of language in the ongoing process of creation, a process that is firmly rooted in the realm of the material, sensual world, and in the immediate concerns and conflicts of life in the Garden.

While Wilkins sought to provide a discursive resolution to the social conflicts in the period by eliminating the subversive threat posed by a dialogical language, Milton, like Donne, suggests that metaphor may serve a socially redemptive function. Milton's own complex and ambiguous poetic practice, which reaches its apogee in *Paradise Lost*, has been identified in a recent study by Sharon Achinstein as part of a systematic poetic strategy for training "revolutionary readers." Because metaphorical complexity confronts readers with their own interpretive agency and choices, it fosters critical and independent thinkers who are capable of analyzing and resisting received political and theological rhetoric, principles, and strategies.[33] The linguistic and intellectual uniformity that is the goal of Wilkins's language projection scheme would no doubt be viewed by the poet as a particularly subtle and insidious form of censorship. The linguistic and sociopolitical order that Wilkins envisions mystifies the material and ideological roots of the English Civil War, betrays the revolutionary principles of the Commonwealth, and creates a nation of servile subjects willing to accede to their own enslavement to a "restored" church and state.

III

In the commitment that they demonstrate to advancing the privileges and power of a patriarchal elite, Wilkins's writings on astronomy and natural philosophy and his language projection scheme are consistent with the dominant ideology of the Royal Society. This nexus of ideological concerns also clearly shapes studies in husbandry undertaken by members of the Royal Society. The science of husbandry was widely viewed as an essential com-

ponent of agrarian improvement schemes in the period. As Andrew
McRae's excellent study on representations of agrarian England
persuasively demonstrates, the rhetoric of agrarian improvement
was embraced to support a broad spectrum of economic and
sociopolitical agendas; while members of the Hartlib Circle had
associated agrarian improvement with social reform, representing it
as a means of addressing the needs of the poor who suffered in
particular the effects of severe food shortages and elevated food
prices in the period, members of the Royal Society saw agrarian
improvement and the science of husbandry as a means of maxi-
mizing the profits of large landholders and enhancing national
power through the creation of a competitive market economy.[34]

Milton's long-standing interest in agriculture is apparent
throughout *Paradise Lost*, as Richard J. DuRocher has argued.[35] Book
8 provides strong indications that Milton values the practical
technical knowledge of husbandry studies far above the abstruse
scientific speculation associated with astronomy in the dialogue
between Adam and Raphael. Together with book 9, it also demon-
strates, however, Milton's resistance to the ideological and material
goals advanced by the husbandry studies of the Royal Society and
suggests that Milton's ideological affinities align him much more
closely with the reformist agenda advanced by the husbandry studies
of the Hartlib circle in the Interregnum.

Milton's dedication of his 1644 treatise on educational and social
reform "Of Education" may in fact signal his sympathy with the
goals of the agrarian reform movement spearheaded by Hartlib and
associates such as Walter Blith and Gabriel Plattes. In Milton's
outline of a "virtuous and noble education," studies of the "authors
of agriculture," including Cato, Varro, and Columella, are to be
preceded only by the study of grammar. Studying these texts would,
Milton reasons, provide students with practical knowledge, "inciting
and enabling them hereafter to improve the tillage of their country,
to recover the bad soil and to remedy the waste that is made of

good," while also rendering them "capable to read any compendious method of natural philosophy." While astronomy, together with arithmetic, geometry, and geography, also occupies a fundamental place in the curriculum, Milton devotes more attention to acknowledging the benefits that students might glean from exposure to the "helpful experiences" of common laborers, of "hunters, fowlers, fishermen, shepherds, gardeners and apothecaries," among others.[35] Milton also takes particular pains to reflect upon the value of the pastoral tradition in English poetry. The poet's early pastoral "L'Allegro," as Michael Wilding has observed, calls attention to the "hardship of physical rural labour, of the need for rest, of the harshness of the places of rest available to the labourer." *Paradise Lost*, like "Of Education" and "L'Allegro," demonstrates Milton's abiding concern with the material conditions of agrarian production and labor in England, and his sympathy with both the common laborer and the yeoman farmer.[36]

In contrast to the programs for agrarian reform and improvement advanced by members of the Hartlib circle during the Interregnum, which were cast as remedies for the suffering of the poor who faced severe food shortages, members of the Royal Society represent their studies in husbandry as advancing the wealth of large landowners and of natural power by revitalizing a competitive market economy. In the dedicatory epistle to Cromwell that prefaces *The English Improver Improved, or The Survey of Husbandry Surveyed* (1649), Walter Blith, a close associate of Hartlib, portrays entrepreneurs in the wool industry as "oppressors" of the poor who are barely able to eke their subsistence from the ravaged soil. Blith and Hartlib both voice their commitments to making their works widely available; Hartlib describes himself as "a conduit-pipe . . . towards the Public," and Blith explains that he writes in "our own naturall Country Language, and in our ordinary and usuall home-spun tearmes" so that his writings would be "clear to each apprehension" and to ensure that "the poorest and plainest Subject" would benefit from his work."[37] Robert Sharrock, a member of the Royal Society, signals his ideological distance from Hartlib and company by asserting in his dedicatory epistle to Boyle that he will not, in "imitation of Some Modern Alchymist, for ostentation bid [the reader] goe, and by the improvement (which I hope may be some of most Readers) be charitable to the poor: Hoping, that for Gods sake they will rather (as they are bound by Obligations inifitely more high) be thereto moved." The needs—let alone the rights—of the poor merit no further discussion from Sharrock, who goes on to dispense advice to the gentleman farmer on the means of maximizing crop production. In *Sylva, or A Discourse on Forest-Trees, and the Propagation of Timber in His Majesties Dominions* (1664), one of the best-known texts on husbandry in the second half of the century, John Evelyn, anxious not to insult the "capacities" of his readers, explains that though he includes a glossary of terms he "did not altogether compile this *Work* for the sake of our *Ordinary Rustics*, but for the more *Ingenious;* the benefit and diversions of *Gentlemen* and Persons of *Quality,* who often refresh themselves in these agreeable *Toiles* of *Planting* and the *Gardens.*" If *Sylva* is, in part, a response to wide-scale deforestation, the work is principally concerned with the industrial uses of timber, which he outlines for each individual species.[38]

Boyle prefaces his discussion of husbandry in *Some Considerations Touching the Usefulness of Experimental Natural Philosophy* (1663) by signaling his ideological distance from Hartlib's strategies for agrarian reform and his own commitment to serving and protecting the rights of the landed elite. While "Physick" or natural philosophy has until recently been necessarily absorbed in "defend[ing] [man] against Revolts and Insurrections at home," it is now prepared, Boyle suggests, to address the real business of contributing to the "Inlargement of [man's] Power over the other Creatures . . . and extend[ing] the Limits of his Empire abroad." In a subsequent section on the usefulness of natural philosophy for the advancement of trade, his comments on sugar production in Barbados illuminate the role that Boyle envisions for husbandry in extending the profitability of the British empire. Boyle invokes the credible witness of an "Ancient Magistrate of that Island" attesting to the astounding levels of productivity on a island estimated to be "short of thirty miles in length." In the interest of establishing the immense productivity of the land, Boyle estimates that the number of "Slaves . . . imploy'd almost totally about the planting of Sugar Canes and making of Sugar amount at least to between five and twenty and thirty thousand persons."39 He offers these collective figures to his gentleman reader so "that you may see how Lucriferous in that place this so recent art of making sugar is, not onely to private men, but to the publick." The irony of the surplus *r* in the adjective Boyle chooses to describe this enterprise would not have been lost on all seventeenth-century readers. Milton was, I believe, capable of perceiving the relationship between the exploitation of laborers in England and in the colonies. If Boyle and Milton share an enthusiasm for agricultural improvement and more generally for applied science and technology, these sciences, in Boyle's mind, become instruments for strengthening the power of the landed elite, for the globalization of English commerce, and for the development of an empire presided over by godly Englishmen.

The misogynist rhetoric that permeates the writings of the Royal Society reinforces an agenda of colonialist expansion. In a passage that immediately follows the one above, Boyle employs a conventional trope, which assumes particular significance in the context of his discussion of the uses of husbandry in enhancing the productivity of colonial holdings. Boyle implicitly conflates the enslaved inhabitants of the colonies with an aggressive, feminized nature to establish an ideological and psychological imperative for the colonialist enterprise, and the experimental philosophy that serves it: "As tis the skilful Diver's work, not onely to gather Pearls and Coral that grew at the bottom of the Sea, and still lay conceal'd there, but also to recover shipwrack'd Goods, that lay buried in the Seas that swallowed them up; so tis the work of the Experimental Philosopher, not onely to dive into the deep Recesses of Nature, and thence fetch up her hidden Riches."[40] In Boyle's account, the material wealth and "Goods" of the New World, implicitly equated with the phallus, are the originary possessions of the colonialist experimental philosopher but have been "swallowed" up by feminized Nature, a seductive and smothering mother who alternately promises and withholds erotic and material satisfaction. The recuperation of the lost material wealth and virility of the colonialist-virtuoso can be effected only through an aggressive assault upon the body of Nature and, implicitly, upon the indigenous peoples of the "New World."

The uneasy relationship between the material and theological goals of his experimental natural philosophy inform Boyle's convoluted construction of feminized Nature in *The Excellency of Theology as Compar'd to Natural Philosophy* and the compromising portrait he erects of the natural philosopher. Boyle defends the piety of the natural philosopher by forcefully affirming the subordination of Nature to Scripture, and in so doing, he invokes the eroticized body of Nature:

Those who make Natural Philosophy their *Mistres*, will probably be the less offended to find her in this Tract represented, if not as an *Handmaid* to Divinity, yet as a Lady of a Lower Rank; because the Inferiority of the Study of Nature is maintain'd by a Person, who, even whilst he asserts it, continues (if not as a Passionate) an Assiduous Courtier of Nature: So that, as far as his Example can reach, it may show, that as on the one side a man need not be acquainted with, or unfit to relish the Lessons taught us in the Book of the Creatures, to think them less Excellent than those, that may be learned in the Book of Scriptures; so on the other side, the Preference for this last Book is very consistent with an high Esteem and an Assiduous Study of the first.[41]

Boyle's representation of the feminized figure of "Divinity" reverberates with images of the idealized lady of Petrarchan verse; the experimentalist-courtier's service to her becomes the vehicle for his own spiritual realization and social aggrandizement. Her social status is a marker of her sexual chastity and of her moral, spiritual, and epistemological reliability. The natural philosopher's service to the lesser lady, however, is implicitly, albeit anxiously, eroticized in Boyle's reference to her as "Mistress" and in his description of the courtier as, at the very least, "assiduous," "if not . . . Passionate." If as a "Lady of a Lower Rank" she is a more available object, whether for marriage or a mutually beneficial sexual dalliance, as a mere "Handmaid," within the material sexual economy of Restoration culture, her low social status marks her as a legitimate target for sexual exploitation by the gentleman virtuoso. Though Boyle tempers the sexual overtones of the natural philosopher's "relish" for the lesser lady by collapsing her body back into text, rhetorically demoted here from the Book of Nature to the "Book of Creatures," her title reinscribes her diminished status as the object of carnal desire. For Boyle, the subordinate and supplementary status of nature to Scripture valorizes as divine and absolute truth the models of sociopolitical order that the natural philosopher locates in nature, while it legitimates the use of applied sciences that transform Second Scripture into a material resource that enhances the wealth—and in so doing, affirms the virility, the social, and ironically, the moral status—of the English gentleman.

IV

Milton's vitalism, as studies by Christopher Hill, Stephen Fallon, and more recently John Rogers have suggested, serves as a crucial marker of his radical politics, of his ideological distance from the orthodox theology of the Anglican Church and, implicitly, from the dominant ideologies of the Royal Society.[42] Though Rogers finds evidence in *Paradise Lost* of the poet's ambivalence toward the radically inclusive model of political order widely associated with vitalism, Milton's representations of a feminized earth that both impregnates and gives birth to itself provide evidence, as Rogers himself notes, of the poet's commitment to decentralized models of power, his reverence for the natural world, and, as I will argue, his willingness to scrutinize and complicate the hierarchy of the sexes. Eve's submissive departure from the scene at the beginning of the dialogue in book 8 provides an ambiguous commentary on women's exclusion from the all-male circles of debate that shaped and authorized representations and interpretations of nature and the body in the period. Eve's absence certainly reflects the limited scope of women's education during the period and women's exclusion from the university and from authorized representations and interpretations of nature.[43] Though the members of the Royal Society legitimated their findings in part by characterizing the laboratory space as open, it was in fact as closed to women as the alchemist's laboratory had been, and perhaps more adamantly so.[44]

The admiring glances that mark Eve's departure from the scene would undoubtedly have been viewed by seventeenth-century women readers such as Margaret Cavendish as small compensation for their exclusion from what was rapidly to become a powerful arena of cultural production in England. The lines that serve ostensibly to affirm Eve's fitness for intellectual activity are, at best, ambivalent. "Yet went she not, as not with such discourse / Delighted," writes Milton of Eve's retreat toward the flower beds, "or not capable her ear / Of what was high" (48–50). While the tortuous syntax and proliferating negatives in these lines may be seen as reflective of the poet's conflicted views of women, they may also be read as inviting the reader to enter into the debates surrounding the appropriate spheres of knowledge and inquiry for women in the period. More query than conclusion, the question itself marks the poet's ideological distance from the exclusively and adamantly all-male Royal Society. The lines encourage the reader to scrutinize the broader role that gender plays in shaping the theory and practices of Restoration natural philosophy and astronomy.

While women's intellectual inferiority and identification with a feminized natural world ostensibly justifies the exclusion of women from participation in the Royal Society, at the beginning of book 8 Eve, rather than Adam, embodies the model of socially responsible science. If, as a number of critics have noted, it is Eve's curiosity about the structure of the universe at the end of book 4 that serves as the catalyst for Adam's cosmological queries, while Adam pursues the speculative science of astronomy, Eve dedicates herself to cultivating the plant life of the garden, to learning and applying the science of husbandry. As Diane McColley notes, Eve embodies an ethic of environmental stewardship, and that stewardship, I wish to add, is explicitly conceived of as maternal.[45] "Her nursery," her careful "tendance" of the "fruits and flowers," which she rather than Adam has named, is valorized as an alternative to the ethos of patriarchal domination that underlies Adam's astronomical speculations. If Eve's identification with nature in *Paradise Lost* may be seen as reinforcing the ages-old association of women and nature, men and culture, it may also be seen as uniquely qualifying her in book 8 to participate responsibly in modes of cultural production that impinge upon the natural world. Milton avoids, however, essentializing Eve's identification with nature by transforming her at the beginning of book 9 into an entrepreneurial farmer whose rhetoric of agrarian improvement—and exploitation—strongly echoes that of the Royal Society.

In book 8, Adam's astronomical speculations, as a number of critics have argued, are ideologically loaded.[46] His privileging of the Copernican over the Ptolemaic model rests upon his belief that the king and nobles exist to be served by their subjects, husbands by their wives:

> this Earth a spot, a grain,
> An Atom, with the Firmament compar'd
> And all her number'd Stars, that seem to roll

Spaces incomprehensible . . .
. . . merely to officiate light
Round this opacous Earth, this punctual spot,
One day and night; in all thir vast survey
Useless besides; reasoning I oft admire,
How Nature wise and frugal could commit
Such disproportions, with superfluous hand
So many nobler Bodies to create,
Greater so manifold to this one use,
For aught appears, and on thir Orbs impose
Such restless revolution day by day
Repeated, while the sedentary Earth,
That better might with far less compass move,
Serv'd by more noble than herself, attains
Her end without least motion, and receives,
As Tribute such a sumless journey brought. (17–20, 22–36)

The sun, figured here as celestial monarch, should, Adam reasons, be served by the subordinate and conspicuously feminized earth. The ideology that shapes Adam's preference for heliocentrism here closely parallel the ideology that informs Wilkins's argument for heliocentrism in his *Discourse*:

The appearances would be the same, in respect of us, if only this little point of Earth were made the subject of these motions, as if the vast Frame of the World, with all those stars of such number and bignes were moved about it. 'Tis a common Maxime, Nature do's nothing in vaine, but in all her courses do's take the most compendious way. 'Tis not therefore (I say) likely, that the whole Fabricke of the Heavens, which do so much exceed our Earth in magnitude and perfection, should be put to undergoe so great and constant a worke in the service of our Earth, which might more easily save all that labour by the circumvolution of it's owne Body, especially, since the Heavens doe not by this motion attaine any farther perfection for themselves, but are made thus serviceable to this little Ball of Earth.

The hierarchical order of English society serves, for Wilkins, as the model for cosmological order. Insofar as the heavens occupy a superior place in the cosmological order, they would not, Wilkins suggests, be made "serviceable" to the lesser earth. Elsewhere, in the *Discovery,* Wilkins invokes woman's "natural" subordination to man to substantiate his assumptions concerning cosmological order. Wilkins draws support for his assertion that the feminized moon "hath not any light but what is bestowed by the Sun" by asserting that "this light" is not in fact *"proper* to the Moone." Wilkins proceeds to explain the *"Aurora* of the Moone" as a "kind of blushing light, that the Sunne causes when he is neere his rising"; this nocturnal encounter between the evidently chaste Moon and the sexually potent Sun also serves to conveniently explain why "waters" sometimes "appeare very red."[47] The sexual passivity that Wilkins assigns to the feminized moon contrasts to the agency that Raphael will attribute to the feminized earth in his response to Adam's speculations. Wilkins invokes aristocratic and patriarchal privilege as supplying crucial ideological support for his modeling of cosmological order; these constructions of cosmological order threaten in turn to naturalize these privileges. Wilkins's seemingly "progressive" support for scientific discovery is pressed into an ideological reading of heliocentrism that provides divine sanction for the oppression of women and the exploitation of the laboring masses.

Raphael's responses to Adam's astronomical speculation suggests that Milton is concerned not with the "correctness" of scientific models for their own sake but rather with the attempts of Wilkins and other members of the Royal Society to assert an interpretive monopoly over the book of nature, and with the specific ideologies their readings would authorize. Raphael responds to Adam's cosmological queries by challenging the ideologies that underlie Adam's preference for heliocentrism and that inform the investigative practices and concerns of the Royal Society:

> consider first, that Great
> Or Bright infers not Excellence: the Earth
> Though, in comparison of Heav'n, so small,
> Nor glistering, may of solid good contain
> More plenty than the Sun that barren shines,
> Whose virtue on itself works no effect,
> But in the fruitful Earth; there first receiv'd
> His beams, unactive else, thir vigor find.
> Yet not to Earth are those bright Luminaries
> Officious, but to thee Earth's habitant. (90–99)

The earth is implicitly associated in the passage with both woman and commoner. The "sun that barren shines" is suggestive at once of monarchical and aristocratic luxury, and of the new wealth of the capitalist entrepreneur, while the "solid good" of the earth implicitly evokes the virtues of the simple yeoman and laboring masses. Raphael's assertion that "Great / Or Bright infers not Excellence" directly refutes the central conviction that informs all of Wilkins's works, that social status is a reliable measure of moral standing. For Milton, political power and social status signify virtue only insofar as they are used to advance the common good. In line 96 the "fruitful Earth" assumes a particularly feminine character. While the passage assigns primary agency to the sun, which confers "his" beams upon the feminized earth, the lines nevertheless foreground the contribution of the feminine principle in the process of sexual generation. The model of political interdependency and Christian *caritas* that Raphael advances undermines attempts to naturalize the privileges of a patriarchal elite and challenges the logic of domination and exploitation that prevails in the postlapsarian world.[48] More broadly, the passage challenges the the elitist ideology

of the Royal Society, which encourages the populace to defer inter-
pretive agency to qualified readers who mystify contentious positions
and transform them into unassailable truths.

V

As a number of critics have noted, Milton's integration of labor
into the prelapsarian world implicitly critiques the life of patrician
luxury while it dignifies labor. The ample periods of rest that punc-
tuate the labors of Adam and Eve serve as a critical counterpoint to
the harsh conditions to which laborers in seventeenth-century England
were subjected. As a model of an ecologically sound applied science
and of engaged and integrated labor, Eve's loving attention to the
fruits and flowers in book 8 is implicitly contrasted to the capitalist
ethos of agrarian improvement that she espouses at the beginning of
book 9. In book 9 Eve's single-minded obsession with maximizing
the profitability of the Garden serves as an essential precondition
for the Fall, while her arguments for the division of labor invoke the
specter of the postlapsarian economy of Restoration England, which
is dependent on the oppression of both the worker and nature:

> *Adam*, well may we labor still to dress
> This Garden, still to tend Plant, Herb and Flow'r,
> Our pleasant task enjoin'd, but till more hands
> Aid us, the work under our labor grows,
> Luxurious by restraint; what we by day
> Lop overgrown, or prune, or prop, or bind,
> One night or two with wanton growth derides
> Tending to wild. Thou therefore now advise
> Or hear what to my mind first thoughts present,
> Let us divide our labors, thou where choice
> Leads thee, or where most needs, whether to wind
> The Woodbinde round this Arbor, or direct

The clasping Ivy where to climb, while I
In yonder Spring of Roses intermixt
With Myrtle, find what to redress till Noon. (9:205–19)

The logic that impel Eve's strategies for agrarian "improvement" in
this passage is that of the entrepreneurial farmer and capitalist. The
adversarial relationship that Eve evokes between humans and nature
in her reference to the "wanton growth" that "derides / Tending to
wild" anticipates the relationship of mankind to a fallen nature. In
the postlapsarian world, moreover, the fate of a suspect nature sub-
jected to an aggressive program of "improvement" is inextricably
tied to that of the worker; the exploitation of both is evoked by the
image of "clasping Ivy" that Eve would have Adam "direct." If
Adam's response to Eve affirms woman's distinct responsibilities in
the domestic sphere—and the ethos of frugality prevalent in domestic
conduct manuals in the period—in asserting that "nothing lovelier
can be found / In Woman, than to study household good" (232–33),
his subsequent observations offers a pointed challenge to the exploita-
tive practices of large landowner:

not so strictly hath our Lord impos'd
Labor as to debar us when we need
Refreshment, whether food, or talk between,
Food of the mind, or this sweet intercourse
Of looks and smiles, for smiles from Reason flow,
To brute deni'd, and are of Love the food,
Love not the lowest end of human life.
For not to irksome toil, but to delight
He made us, and delight to Reason join'd.
These paths and Bowers doubt not but our joint hands
Will keep from Wilderness with ease, as wide
As we need walk, till younger hands ere long
Assist us. (9:235–47)

While animal-rights activists would have much to take issue with here, the passage invokes the hierarchical relationship between humans and animals to argue against hierarchies among men. The lines implicitly indict the exploitation of workers who are reduced to beasts of burden. In referring to the laborers who will ultimately supplement and displace himself and Eve as "younger hands," Adam implicitly invokes the model of the small family farm as the basis for the Edenic economy. Unlike Eve, who is of course about to fall prey to the serpent and a logic of domination that will disrupt every facet of creation, Adam demonstrates little concern with beating back the wilderness. In these lines Milton demonstrates his awareness of the extent to which the rhetoric of agrarian "improvement" is increasingly invoked to enhance the wealth and privilege of the landed elite. Together books 8 and 9 extend Milton's critique of the coercive ideology evident in Wilkins's astronomical works into a broader ideological and environmental critique of the theories and practices of the Royal Society.

If in book 9 Eve serves as the spokesperson for an ethic of environmental exploitation, she is repeatedly identified with nature throughout the epic. In book 8 Adam's relationship to Eve and to nature are represented as inextricably implicated in one another. Eve is described as

> Not obvious, not obtrusive, but retir'd,
> The more desirable, or to say all;
> Nature herself, though pure of sinful thought,
> Wrought in her so. (504–7)

If "Nature herself" is the subject of "wrought in her so" and suggests the agency of "Nature" operating upon Eve, the phrase "though pure of sinful thought" indicates that Eve is also identified as "Nature herself." In this passage, the negation that defines the purity of both Eve and nature anticipates the Fall and, more immediately,

Adam's reactionary response to the attractiveness of both of these feminized figures. The angel resists Adam's attempts to attribute corruption to Eve / nature and implicitly whatever strategies Adam might be formulating for their rehabilitation. The cautionary lecture that the angel delivers to Adam on the dangers of deferring his own judgment before Eve may be read as insisting upon both the primacy of Scripture over nature and the importance of preserving one's own interpretive and moral agency. Though Adam deems Eve, as the embodiment of the Book of Nature, as "in outward / Elaborate, of inward less exact" (588–89), he nevertheless confesses that he is sorely tempted to accept her as an appropriate guide for his own actions; in his judgment the "Wisdom" that she supplies surpasses all other forms of knowledge:

> Her loveliness, so absolute she seems
> And in herself complete, so well to know
> Her own, that what she wills to do or say,
> Seems wisest, virtuousest, discreetest, best,
> All higher knowledge in her presence falls
> Degraded, Wisdom in discourse with her
> Looses discount'nanc't, and like folly shows;
> Authority and Reason on her wait. (547–54)

Adam's elevation of Eve's judgment over his own, and over that of God and angel, suggests the consequences of privileging the authority of readings of the Book of Nature over Scripture, and the dangers of elevating any human authority over that of the "inner light," the voice of God within. The loss of self-control that Adam feels in elevating Eve / nature above God leads him to construct "her" as fallen, as "degrad[ing]" "all higher knowledge." Adam transforms his desire for Eve into an argument for his suppression of her. Though in book 12 Adam characterizes Eve as a "fair defect" of nature, at once damning both nature and herself, in book 8 his incipient condemnation of Eve—and implicitly of nature as well—elicits the angel's reprobation: "Accuse not nature, she hath done her part" (61). While the passage effectively guards against the exploitation of Second Scripture by insisting on man's direct and unmediated access to the divine by means of the inner light, it might also be read as reinscribing Eve's subordinate status within the gendered hierarchy of the companionate marriage. If Milton enlarges the spheres for women's participation in modes of cultural production in book 8 and acknowledges their active participation in the English economy, he nevertheless privileges Adam's access to the "inner light" over Eve's. Whether he does so out of a politic awareness of the contention surrounding claims to women's equality, as Wilding has argued, or out of his own intimate and anxious understanding of the revolutionary implications of the doctrine of the inner light, must remain, I believe, an open question.[49] What is more certain, however, is that the agency that Milton affords both Eve and the feminized natural world considerably exceeds and contests the bounds imposed by the members of the Royal Society.

Adam's astronomical speculations, which Milton characterizes at the beginning of book 8 as "studious thoughts abtruse"(40), distance Adam from Eve, and implicitly from nature and the immediate concerns of the Garden. The phrase associates astronomy imagistically with the pedantry and isolation of the university. The adjective *abtruse*, which the OED defines as "concealed" or "thrust away," suggests an incipient alienation between Adam and Eve, and between Adam and God. It invokes the shame that follows from the Fall and is associated with the concealment and rejection of the body. Milton implies, then, that the ideology with which he associates astronomy stems from an objectification of and alienation from the body, woman, and nature and as such fosters an ethic of exploitation and domination.

Adam's dialogue with Raphael leads him to conclude that at best astronomy, as a metaphor for speculative science, is a distraction from far more important and immediate concerns:

> That not to know at large of things remote
> From use, obscure and subtle, but to know
> That which before us lies in daily life,
> Is the prime Wisdom; what is more, is fume,
> Or emptiness, or fond impertinence,
> And renders us in things that most concern
> Unpractic'd, unprepar'd, and still to seek. (192–97)

Though Raphael responds to the ideological threat implicit in Adam's cosmological speculations, Adam's summary dismissal of astronomy implicitly associates the science with an ethos of aristocratic leisure and privilege that is identified with the abandonment of a voluntaristic theology, and of applied sciences that foster the well-being of the Garden and its inhabitants. Astronomy is at best, the passage suggests, an evasion of more immediate and material concerns. For Milton, fidelity to God necessarily entails a commitment to addressing and *redressing* the material conditions of everyday life.

If books 8 and 9 provides strong indications that the science of husbandry figures prominently among those sciences that address the most immediate concerns of life in the Garden, it may also be seen as offering a critique of the science as it is pursued by members of the Royal Society. Milton's critique of astronomy in *Paradise Lost* can be read as a rejection of the colonialist ambitions—and more broadly, the ethic of exploitation—that permeate and shape Wilkins's writings on astronomy and Boyle's on husbandry. Balachandra Rajan has argued that *Paradise Lost* is an anti-imperialist epic, observing that Milton identifies Satan's journey with Vasco da Gama's voyage to India, "inscrib[ing] the Satanic voyage within subsequent voyages of exploration and commerce as the tainted origin from which they may need to be rescued."[50] While book 1 associates the material excesses of Pandemonium with the Indian empire, Milton, he argues, subsequently transforms India into a paradise to be plundered. The poet's account of Satan's arrival in the Garden in book 4 may moreover be seen as probing and critiquing the motives that impel the colonialist enterprise. Freshening up from his interplanetary flight, Satan perches on the "verdurous wall of Paradise," "Which to our general sire gave prospect large / Into his nether empire neighboring round"(143–44). Milton's repetition of the word "prospect" within the space of forty lines lends emphasis to the word, which the OED defines alternately as "to look out" and "to work a mine, to test its value, explore region for gold." As Merchant has observed, in book 1 Milton represents mining as a metaphorical rape of the feminized natural world as he refers to the fallen angels who with "impious hands / Rifl'd the bowels of thir mother Earth / For Treasures better hid"(686–88). Looking down into Eden, Satan may lay claim to something like a God's-eye view, but he will never know it as Adam and Eve have.[51] For Satan, Eden is merely an opportunity to be exploited in his quest to satisfy his unbounded ambition, escape his "infinite despair"(4:74). "Which way I fly is Hell; myself am Hell"(4:75), reflects the lost angel moments before he alights in Paradise. If Milton's descriptions of Satan's flight through the heavens reflect the poet's interest in the new astronomy, they also demonstrate the poet's concern, evident throughout book 8, that the theories, practices, and technologies that will be developed under the auspices of the restored monarchy will merely provide more sophisticated tools for domination.

The poet of *Paradise Lost* has come a long way since his days at Cambridge, when he could imagine a day when

At last most of the chances and changes of the world will be so quickly perceived that to him who holds this stronghold of wisdom hardly anything can happen in his life which is unforeseen or fortuitous. He will indeed seem to be one whose rule and dominion the stars obey, to whose command earth and sea hearken, and whom winds and tempests serve; to whom, lastly, Mother Nature herself has surrendered, as if indeed some god had abdicated the throne of the world and entrusted its rights, laws, and administration to him as governor.

Satan's flight to earth and Adam's stargazing are, one suspects, both sardonic reflections on the intellectual hubris that underlay the poet's own youthful enthusiasm for natural philosophy and the role it would play in creating the "New Jerusalem." "Nor should you hesitate, gentlemen," wrote Milton as a student at Cambridge, "to fly into the heavens. . . . Let there be nothing secret from you about the purpose of either Jove or Nature. . . . Not even the tiniest stars should be hidden from you. . . . You must follow the sun on his journey—be his companions and call time itself to a reckoning, and demand an account of its eternal flight. . . . your mind should not consent to be limited and circumscribed by the earth's boundaries, but should range beyond the confines of the world."[52]

    "Heaven is for thee too high / To know what passes there. . . . Dream not of other worlds" (172–75) writes the poet in 1667, acknowledging the consequences of intellectual overreaching combined with the logic of domination and anxious to circumscribe the powers and geographical reach of the restored monarchy. Milton's concerns would be shared by some Americans three centuries later, when funds for the War on Poverty were siphoned off to fund the war in Vietnam and NASA's race for space. They are still relevant today in a nation that has one of the highest infant mortality rates of any industrialized country[53] but annually spends billions on space exploration. In 1667, however, astronomy may yet have been only a metaphor for theories and practices that advanced the privileges of a small but powerful elite who dreamed of extending their empire into even the heavens. Under the restored monarchy, the poet suggests, the very stars will be commodified, "calculate[d]" (80) by individuals who are intoxicated by dreams of power that at best distract them from the Edenic dreams of the Commonwealth, from cultivating the "New Jerusalem" in England.

4

"THE THREATNING ANGEL AND THE SPEAKING ASS"

The Masculine Mismeasure of Madness in Anne Finch's "The Spleen"

Anne Finch's "The Spleen" (1701) provides a critique of the role that masculinist representations of feminized nature and the female body play in justifying the confinement of the upper-class woman within the home and her exclusion from modes of cultural production. In the seventeenth and eighteenth centuries the bodies of women, like those of homosexuals, the lower classes, and the colonized, became "signs" to be incorporated into medical narratives that naturalize and legitimize the privileged position of a masculine elite atop the hierarchies of gender, class, and race. The "Enlightenment axiom that men are by nature equal," as Schiebinger points out, could be overridden by "objective" "scientific" evidence of the "natural inferiority" of women, people of color, and members of the laboring classes.[1] This repressive ideology, however, also generated (m)odes of resistance. "The Spleen" recognizes that late seventeenth-century medical narratives simply reconstruct existing conceptions of feminine instability evident in the works of male poets from Sidney onward under the aegis of a new narrative authority.[2]

As both Barbara McGovern and Charles Hinnant and have observed, Finch's interest in the discourses of "the spleen," and of "hysteria" and "melancholy" was far from academic.[3] Finch's struggle against painful and debilitating symptoms that were variously identified within these discursive categories is reflected in a number of her poems. McGovern, in an effort to affirm the physiological

roots of Finch's suffering, has suggested that the poet would in fact
be classifiable in contemporary psychiatric discourse as manic-
depressive.[4] It is somewhat ironic and certainly illustrative of the
dynamic nature of medical and scientific discourse that patients
diagnosed in 1992 as "manic-depressive" are, in 1997, more likely to
be described as suffering from "bipolar disorder." Equating "the
spleen" too closely with contemporary psychiatric diagnostic cate-
gories runs the risk of mystifying the ideological assumptions that
inhere in these discourses, assumptions that have a very material
impact upon the experience of the individual sufferer, and on the
broader culture, as the debates concerning the discourse of AIDS
have demonstrated in recent years. Assuming that there was in fact a
physiological basis for what Hinnant describes as Finch's "obsessive
preoccupation with melancholy, loss, mourning, care and the
spleen,"[5] it is important to note that in contrast to poems such as
"Ardelia to Melancholy," "The Spleen" is concerned not simply
with the individual experience of psychic pain and emotional
suffering but with medical discourse specifically, and with the
ideologies it both reflects and perpetuates.

   In her critique of the ideology of the spleen, Finch by necessity
adopts—and subverts—the conceptions of "nature," "femininity,"
and "disease" encoded in the discourses of Restoration natural
philosophy, medicine, and poetry, and in the works of Thomas
Sydenham and Abraham Cowley in particular. Finch explores the
contingent claims and methodologies of the Puritan "empirical"
physician and the Royalist poet, popularizer of the Pindaric ode
and author of a well-known ode "To the Royal Society," in order to
unmask the misogynist ideology that both men advance. Finch's ode
neither endorses nor simply opposes the ideology of the spleen, but
rather examines the form and ideology of masculinist science and
poetry as they are implicated in one another. If the open form of
the ode provides Finch with a model for the means through which
patriarchal authority is disseminated, it also embodies the form of

feminized resistance that these strategies engender. In this respect, "The Spleen" demonstrates the dynamic nature of all cultural narratives and the inadequacy of the critical position that constructs a mutable, feminine poetics in opposition to the fixed narratives of a masculinist scientific theory and practice.

I

The Pindaric ode was resurrected in the latter half of the seventeenth century by Cowley, author of a *Proposition for the Advancement of Experimental Philosophy,* "To the *Royal Society,*" a laudatory ode that celebrates natural philosophy as an exclusively "Male Virtue," and "Upon Dr. Harvey," all of which were included in *The Works of Abraham Cowley,* first published posthumously in 1668 and reprinted throughout the century. Cowley, who received an M.D. at Oxford in 1657 and who became an active member of the Royal Society with its foundation in 1662, is representative of the emerging role of the physician-experimentalist that was the legacy of William Harvey. Harvey, who is best known for his description of the circulation of the blood, advocated an experimental approach to medicine that would inform the methodology of the Royal College of Physicians from the 1640s onward and would eventually play an important role in shaping the experimental interests of the Royal Society.[6] Cowley's "Ode upon Dr Harvey" celebrates Harvey's achievement as emblematic of the progressive control that experimental philosophy will achieve over feminized nature and the body.

Finch's identification of the open form of the "Pindaric" with the masculinist discourses of medicine and with the contingent claims and methodologies of the physician-virtuoso of the Royal Society has some precedent. The ideas reflected in the Pindaric ode, as practiced by Cowley in particular, were thought, as David Trotter has observed, to arise from the "possibly fortuitous external relations between sense impressions," rather than simply reflecting a preconceived argument or traditional "truths."[7] Trotter notes the similarities between popular descriptions of the Pindaric ode—and more broadly, the aesthetics of "randomness" and "discontinuity" with which it came to be identified—and Sprat's description of experimental method. "The true Experimenting," wrote Thomas Sprat, "has this one thing inseparable from it, never to be a fix'd and settled Art, and never to be limited by constant Rules."[8] Sprat's observation reflects the Royal Society's commitment to an inductive methodology and their rejection of theoretical closure and dog-matism. The Pindaric ode, then, was associated for Sprat and Cowley and, I believe, for Finch with the contingent, voluntaristic method-ology espoused by the English experimentalists. Finch's opening allusion to Cowley's Pindaric "Brutus" signals her desire to position "The Spleen" in relation to Cowley's ode and ideology and reflects her awareness that the flexible methodology and terminology of the physician-virtuoso serves, in fact, to advance a masculinist ideology. In Cowley's traditional rendering of the tale of Brutus's defeat at Philippi, the "*Ill Fate*" that causes the hero's defeat presents itself in the form of a "Spright," taking him by surprise at Philippi:

> Nor durst it in *Philippi's* field appear,
>> But *unseen* attaqu'ed thee there.
> Had it presum'ed in any shape thee to oppose,
> Thou wouldst have forc'ed it back upon thy foes. (58–61)

In revising Cowley's narrative to indicate that Brutus is "vanquish'd by the *Spleen*," Finch suggests that the methodological flexibility and mutable discourse of "the spleen" plays a crucial role in dissemi-nating a masculinist ideology represented by the male physician and virtuoso. Her allusion to Brutus as a victim of the spleen feminizes him, transforming him from a heroic subject to a self-defeating object of medical scrutiny. He becomes a victim of the physician's will to power, which is masked by claims to ideological neutrality.

At the same time, however, the allusive form of Finch's own critique reflects the poet's determination to work within the Protean methodology and discourse of "the spleen" in order to undermine it. Ironically, Finch's critique confers new meaning on Cowley's apology for Brutus, in which he exhorts the reader to join in resisting tyranny:

> Can we stand by and see
> Our *Mother* robb'ed, and bound, and ravisht be,
>   Yet not to her assistance stir,
> Pleas'd with the *Strength* and *Beauty* of the *Ravisher.* (32–35)

Finch's incorporation of the story of Brutus's denial at Phillipi into her own narrative of "The Spleen" is consistent with the central project of the poem: to appropriate and transform masculine myths and the modes of discourse through which these social myths are shaped. Ironically, the only antidote for the spleen is the spleen itself.

In his account of Cowley's life that prefaced the 1668 edition and subsequent editions of Cowley's poems, Thomas Sprat, historian of the Royal Society and Cowley's close associate and literary executor, distinguishes Cowley's Pindaric as an expressly masculine verse form. Responding to those "Admirers of Gentleness without sinews," who responded uneasily to the irregular meter and somewhat random argumentative structure of the ode, Sprat argued that "there is a kind of variety of Sexes in Poetry as well as in Mankind: that as the peculiar excellence of that Feminine kind, is smoothnesse and beauty: so strength is the chief praise of the masculine."[9] The "roughness" of Cowley's meter and argument are, for Sprat, distinctly masculine attributes.

Cowley's own reflections on the Pindaric undoubtedly fostered this view of it as a distinctly masculine verse form. In a footnote to "The Praise of Pindar," the poet describes the ode as a "bold, free, enthusiatical kind of Poetry, as of men inspired by *Bacchus*, that is,

Half-Drunk." The description differs markedly from the standard by which Cowley measures the poetry of Katherine Anne Philips. In his poem "*On the death of Mrs.* Katherine Philips," the "poetic" virtues that Cowley lauds are those associated with the conventional feminine virtues of restraint and moral purity. Philips's wit is, Cowley suggests, thankfully tempered by her "virtue," for

> . . . Wit's like a Luxurian Vine;
>> Unless to Virtue's prop it joyn,
>> Firm and Erect towards Heaven bound;
> Though it with beauteous Leaves, and pleasant Fruit be crown'd,
> It lies deform'd, and rotting on the ground. (69–72)

The feminine virtues that are canonized in Phillips are a rod with which to beat those female poets who, like Behn, might not so willingly submit their vines for binding, and would dare present their "deform'd" and "rotting" fruits before the public eye. Finch's admiration for Behn is evident in "The Circuit of Appollo," in which Apollo observes of Behn that there "was not on the earth / Her superiour in fancy, in language, or witt." If Apollo qualifies his praise by observing that "A little too loosely she writt," the line seems a rather obligatory and cursory concession to public propriety on Finch's part. Verbal echoes of Behn's ideal of a free sexual economy in "The Golden Age" inform Finch's Edenic description of sexual experience prior to the regulatory discourse of "the spleen." In "The Introduction" Finch voices her suspicion of the ideals of feminine submissiveness and passivity that Cowley, among others, enshrines in Philips. The woman poet, Finch suggests, must be content with obscurity—or at least appear as such—or else "be dispis'd, aiming to be admir'd." "The Spleen," like "The Intro-duction," reflects Finch's concern with the creative autonomy of woman.[10] The "bold" and "free" verse that for Cowley marks the highest achievement of the male poet, when undertaken by a woman,

Finch suggests, can only be read as a sign of the pathological ambition that the medical discourse of Sydenham and company would cure.

II

If Finch's choice of the Pindaric reflects her desire to examine the form and ideology of the spleen as implicated in one another, the public form of the Pindaric also seems a particularly appropriate medium for treating a phenomenon that was viewed, from the late seventeenth century onward, as peculiarly English.[11] The spleen, moreover, was a "disease" associated specifically with the upper classes and with a sedentary life of luxury. In this respect, as John Mullan among others has emphasized, the spleen marked not simply affliction but also privilege.[12] The terms "hysteric" and "hypochondriack" might be used to distinguish between female and male "sufferers" respectively. Referring implicitly to the male sufferer, Sydenham asserted that splenetic individuals were given to "impetuosities of mind," were otherwise "very prudent and judicious," and "excel[led] for deep thought and wisdom of Speech, others whose minds were never excited by these Provocations to thinking." "*Aristotle,*" he concluded, was in the right when he said that "Melancholy people were most ingenious."[13] This conception of "the spleen" was to be reinforced throughout the eighteenth century.[14] The "spleen," as Markley has observed, was increasingly seen to mark the heightened sensibility or "moral sensitivity" of the gentleman. The symptoms of the spleen, Markley argues, were less frequently invoked by members of the aristocracy than by writers interested in advancing their social status.[15] For the male writer, at least, displays of splenetic symptomatology became a means of affirming or enhancing social, political, and intellectual authority. The discourse of the spleen, Finch implies, legitimates "scientifically" the claims of upper-class men to power and privilege.

While the symptoms of the spleen or hysteria confirm the "femininity" and delicacy of the upper-class woman, they also undermine her claim to intellectual equality and justify her confinement to and subordination within the private space of the home. Though by the end of the seventeenth century the direct attribution of "hysteria" to the womb was being called into question, hysteria continued to be a peculiarly female disturbance. Descriptions of nervous disorders in the early works of Sydenham, Thomas Willis, and Bernard de Mandeville continue to reflect patriarchal myths concerning the limited intellectual capabilities of women and the excesses and inherent corruption of woman's sexuality. Thomas Willis observes the frequency with which his contemporaries in the medical profession wrongly "accuse the evil influence of the womb," suggesting that the "Womb is for the most part"—though by no means entirely—guiltless." Hysteria, for Willis, is also caused by the "weak Constitution of the Brain and *Genus Nervosum*."[16] Late seventeenth- and eighteenth-century physiologists would, in fact, broaden the locus of feminine pathology to include the entire body. Measured against the anatomically determined physical, intellectual, and moral perfection of the upper-class male, the physical, intellectual, and moral weakness and deviance of the upper-class woman becomes an argument for her circumscribed domestic existence and necessitates continued strategies for protecting and controlling her.

The question with which Finch opens her poem, "What art thou SPLEEN which ev'rything dost ape?," defines her central concern with the flexibility of the discourse of the spleen and with the semiotics of disease. Finch's question is, I believe, a direct response to Sydenham's writings on "Hypochondriack and Hysterick Diseases." "Hysteria," writes Sydenham, is "so strangely various, that it resembles almost all the Diseases poor Mortals are inclined to; for in whatever part it seats itself, it presently produces such Symptoms as belong to it."[17] While Finch's question may be seen as simply reinforcing Sydenham's conception of "hysteria," it may also be seen as probing the political uses of a discourse that can be infinitely adaptable to the ideological interests served by the male diagnostician.

If the writings of both Sydenham and Cowley reflect common assumptions about gender, in other respects their ideological commitments were distinctly at odds. In contrast to Cowley, who was a Royalist and a member of the Royal Society, Sydenham, who had fought on the Parliamentary side in the Civil War, was a staunch Whig who ran for Parliament on two separate occasions. Andrew Cunningham has observed that the motivations Sydenham cites for his medical studies in a work of 1665 demonstrate his persistent commitment to the reformist goals associated with Puritan millenarianism. Whether he was barred from participating or simply chose not to join, Sydenham's staunch adherence to the republican ideals of the Commonwealth likely account for his apparently never being a member of the Royal Society. Sydenham's emphasis on observation and experience over theoretical formulations nevertheless mark affinities with the practices of the Royal Society. Sydenham himself attributes his commitment to an empirical methodology to the influence of Robert Boyle, whose residence in Oxford from 1654 to 1656 was "opposite All Souls College, where Sydenham lived until 1656." Cunningham has documented numerous avenues of possible contact between Boyle and Sydenham, noting that in London, Sydenham was to become a next-door neighbor to Lady Ranelagh, with "whom Boyle often visited and with whom he was eventually to live." Though on the Continent Sydenham's research was highly regarded and Sydenham would eventually come to be known as the "English Hippocrates," during the period in which Finch composed her poem "the advocacy of Sydenhamian medicine was a politically loaded act." In fact, as Cunningham has observed, "any defender of Sydenham was still virtually identifying himself as a supporter of the Good Old Cause (an unpopular position, especially after 1689)."[18] Finch's poem suggests that Henry Stubbe may not have been alone in the connections that he invoked between Sydenham and the Royal

Society, and Boyle in particular. If Stubbe's description of Sydenham as a "semi-virtuoso" was evidently intended as an epithet,[19] on at least one occasion his attack on Boyle took the form of invoking his methodological and implicitly ideological affinities to Sydenham: "I know what any physician may, as the mode is, tell you to your face, but except it be such as Dr. Sydenham and young Coxe, I believe not one lives that doth not condemn your experimental philosophy."[20]

Sydenham, as Cunningham notes, was neither a radical nor a democrat; his primary concern was with the "rights of the *free-holder,* the independent land owner who could 'live off his own.'" Marginalized during the Restoration for his political views, however, and consulting only periodically in cases involving well-to-do patients, Sydenham's practice was primarily composed of poor people, and this factor played a critical role in shaping the approach to epidemiology that is regarded as a Sydenham's distinct and substantial contribution to the history of medicine. University-educated physicians, as Cunningham observes, did not view fevers and other maladies as primary disorders subject to relatively uniform regimens of treatment; rather they viewed a fever, for example, as the manifestation of a preexisting and fundamentally individual disorder in the physical constitution of the patient and held that the identification of this underlying cause was an essential precondition of treatment. "Even if, in the course of an epidemic, a physician should see several cases of the same fever, they were to him different instances because they were in different, individual, patients."[21] This individualistic ethos undoubtedly often had fatal consequences and serves perhaps as a cautionary tale on the productive limits of knowledge that is "local," "situated," and "particular." Based on generalizations drawn almost exclusively from his treatment of the poor, Sydenham's pioneering studies in epidemiology are unimpeded by the ideological imperative to valorize his patients' individuality; in these, he focused on the disease as a distinct and unvarying phenomenon and, through trial and error, devised effective treatments. As disorders that are exclusively manifested, as he observes, in the privileged classes, hypochondria and hysteria remain, however, uniquely resistant to his attempts to confine them—and implicitly, his upper-class patients—within uniform diagnostic categories.

Quite simply,"hypochondriachal and hysterick diseases," remain, by Sydenham's definition, whatever the physician wishes them to be:

A Day would scarce suffice to reckon upon all the Symptoms belonging to Hysterick Diseases, so various are they, and so contrary to one another, that *Proteus* had no more shapes, nor the Chameleon so great Variety of Colours. . . . Nor are they only very various, but also so irregular, that they cannot be contained under any uniform Type, which is unusual in other Diseases, for they are as it were a disorderly heap of *Phaenomena*, so that it is very hard to write the *History of the Disease.*

The failure of the medical establishment to confine the behavior of its masculine sufferers to "any uniform Type" served, for Sydenham and his successors, merely to affirm their individuality and immunity from a deterministic natural law.[22] The resistance that the male sufferer's behavior poses to scientific generalization in itself provides "scientific proof" of his genius, confirms his social position, and safeguards him against challenges to his authority by women and members of the lower classes. At the same time, the discourse of "the spleen" became part of an "ideology of sentiment," which, as Markley argues, naturalizes class distinctions by "implicitly identifying the victims of social inequality"—men, women, and children—with "feminine powerlessness."[23] The ideology of the spleen, and more broadly, of sentimentality, facilitates the dissemination of paternalistic authority in the eighteenth century.

In contrast to the male sufferer, the female sufferer was constitutionally incapable of abiding by natural law; her body was, to the exclusively male medical establishment, inherently disorderly. While, like that of their male counterparts, the behavior of female sufferers also could not "be contained under any uniform type," the discourse of the spleen, as applied to women, and of hysteria and the conceptions of feminine pathology and debility they reinforced, were infinitely expansive. These discourses were capable of describing—and dismissing—the range of possible modes of feminine resistance to masculine domination and domestic confinement, from the depression and resignation suggested by Finch's reference to "a Calm of stupid Discontent" to vocal outbursts of "Storm"-like "rage" (7, 8). If, for Finch, "abused mankind . . . never yet thy real cause could find," it is because the poem represents the causes of the "spleen" as linguistic and ideological; these causes can be explored only through the broader examination she undertakes in the poem of the behavior prescribed within a patriarchal culture and reinforced by its medical representatives.

For Sydenham, hysteria is the natural state of the upper-class woman and is identified with her physical—and implicitly her moral—weakness: "Very few Women, which Sex is half of grown People, are quite free from every assault of this Disease," states Syndenham, "excepting those who [are] accustomed to labour." Though Sydenham prescribes a rugged session of horseback riding for the hypochondriac, noting that "it is very proper for Men, and soonest restores their Health," he suggests that it is less appropriate for women, "who are accustomed to a slothful and delicate way of life" and "may be injured by Motion." If, on the one hand, the upper-class woman is morally culpable for her symptoms, which are a function of her "slothfulness," or as he suggests elsewhere, of her "crude and lax habit of body," he nevertheless suggests that she is biologically designed for inactivity, and, moreover, anatomically incapable of rational thought:

The inward Man consists of a due Series, and as it were a Fabrick of the Spirits, to be viewed only by the Eye of *Reason:* And as this is nearly joyned, and as it were united with a Constitution of the Body, so much the more easily or difficultly the Frame of it is disordered, by how much the constitutive Principles that are allotted us by Nature, are more or less firm: Wherefore this Disease seizes more Women than Men, because kind Nature has bestowed on them a more delicate and fine Habit of Body, having designed them only for an easie Life, and to perform the tender Offices of Love: But she gave to Men robust Bodies, that they might be able to delve and manure the Earth, to kill wild Beasts for Food and the Like.[24]

The "Fabrick of Spirits" can be viewed only "by the Eye of Reason" because, when in proper working order, it is inseparable for Sydenham from reason itself. The passage illustrates the role that "scientific" conceptions of gender played in justifying woman's exclusion from and objectification by the discourses of medicine. Because "the Eye of Reason" is, for woman, in a perpetual blur, she is incapable of deciphering the order in man's body, or the disorder of her own. The passage suggests, then, that for Sydenham, like de Mandeville after him, hysteria is implicitly equated with sexual excess.[25] The "easie life" and confinement of the domestic woman make her easier to keep an eye on, because, after all, her "delicate and fine Habit of Body" and her eagerness to perform her "tender Offices of Love" render her more vulnerable to having her "Fabrick" disordered.

Given the enthusiasm with which Sydenham seems to have recommended the removal of large quantities of blood from his female patients, his treatments may, indeed, have proved quite effective in transforming the diffident and discontented hysteric into something closer to his idealized image of feminine delicacy and docility. Sydenham's writings suggest that his female patients were treated as unreliable witnesses to the effects of his treatments upon their bodies. Strangely, female patients would frequently "think themselves worse" after three or four days of bloodletting; the "despair" they reported experiencing, however, was merely a symptom of the disorder itself. In the one instance of hysterical behavior Sydenham noted in a male patient, the doctor observes that the symptoms appeared to have been brought on by a lengthy fever coupled with bloodlettings, and by being barred from what Sydenham refers to rather ambiguously as "the use of Flesh." Not surprisingly, the patient finds himself reduced to a state of continual crying. Thankfully, he is returned to his natural state of masculine vigor after Sydenham orders the bloodletting halted and, as an antidote for the patient's "Emptiness," prescribes moderate doses of "Flesh" and "wine." If Sydenham is intent on curing the male hysteric of his effeminacy, the condition of woman was chronic and incurable and, with the help of the sympathetic physician, sometimes even fatal.[26]

While Finch's poem, as I have suggested, ultimately implicates both the Royalist experimentalist and the puritan "semivirtuoso" in a shared misogyny, at various points in the poem she nevertheless invokes a long-standing association of "the spleen" with Puritanism:[27]

> Falsly, the Mortal Part we blame
>   Of our deprest and pond'rous Frame,
>   Which, till the First degrading Sin
>   Let Thee [the spleen], its dull Attendant, in,
>   Still with the Other did comply. (26–30).

For Finch it is not the corruption but the denial of the body that accounts for the state of our "deprest and pond'rous Frame." Finch's use of the word "Frame" suggests both the body and the way in which the world is represented by and to us. The "Mortal Part" refers not simply to the body but also to woman, who has been traditionally associated with the material world and with the sexual, corrupt body. The Fall, Finch reminds the reader, stemmed not from the corruption of the body but rather from its compliance with the soul. If sex in Eden was a consensual act, woman nevertheless now bears the moral onus. The "dull Attendant" suggests the function that the discourse of the spleen plays in policing woman's sexuality in a postlapsarian, patriarchal world. Stripped of autonomy and relegated to a state of perfect compliance, woman, Finch suggests, nevertheless continues to be viewed as the source of evil, the originator of all psychosocial ills. The lines implicitly invite Tory resistance to an ideology and medical discourse that she deflects, at least in this passage, onto the albeit embattled proponents of the "Good Old Cause."

In Finch's revisionist narrative of Genesis, the "reign" of the spleen is identified with the Fall, and with the emergence of a patriarchal authority that equates feminine desire with sin and pathology. The discourse of the spleen, then, intensifies the feminine desire it would repress:

> Whilst Man his Paradice possest,
> His fertile Garden in the fragrant East,
> And all united Odours smelt,
> No armed Sweets, until thy Reign,
> Cou'd shock the Sense, or in the Face
> A flusht, unhandsom Colour place.
> Now the *Jonquille* o'ercomes the feeble Brain;
> We faint beneath the Aromatick Pain,
> Till some offensive Scent thy Pow'rs appease,
> And Pleasure we resign for short, and nauseous Ease. (34–43)

"Armed Sweets" refers to the "Jonquilles" and confections that the lover comes bearing; at the same time it suggests that in the repressive culture of the poet, the lover's body is more likely to be feared as debased—or as a potential weapon—than consumed with relish. As it is, any hint of sensuality is regarded as "shock[ing]" because it threatens or defies a social order dependent on the repression of the body; also, because desire always threatens to reveal itself, every encounter seems all the more charged. The coquette's flushed color is deemed "unhandsom" by Finch because it is associated with the repression of desire and compliance with masculine authority. At the same time, she recognizes that others might find it "unhandsom" precisely because it betrays the coquette's underlying desire. Finch's ostensible acknowledgment of feminine debility—"We faint beneath the Aromatick Pain"—is rather a description of the body in the throes of desire. As Mullan notes, "The distinction between the flush of an improper excitement and the virtuous blush of an entranced sensibility is a difficult and shifting one." The threat posed by the coquette's desire is neutralized by her reduction to hysteric, and she is punished, relates Finch, repeating Sydenham's adjective, by the "offensive" onslaught of the smelling salts. The military motif in the passage echoes Sydenham, who recommends that "If the *Disease* be such . . . that it will not bear a Truce . . . we must presently use Hysterick Medicines which by their strong and noisom Smell, recall the exorbitant and deserting Spirits to their proper Stations."[28] In Finch's scenario, the woman, punished for if not purged of her desires, surrenders her intellectual and sexual autonomy for an easy—and nauseating—life, assuming her "proper station" as a delicate, domesticated creature. In condemning the discourse of the spleen as an extension of the Puritan ideology with which Sydenham's writings are associated, Finch simultaneously undermines the misogynist rhetoric and ideology that serves as a crucial tool for advancing the authority of the Royal Society.

The role of the masculinist ideology of the spleen in regulating and containing female sexuality is evident in Finch's portrait of the coquette whose seductiveness is permissible only as a display of helplessness and debility. "Assum[ing] a soft, a melancholy Air" (103), displaying her sensitivity—and her symptomatology—the coquette reduces herself to a passive portrait, an object of art, surrendering "Sense," both mind and sensuality, to allow "the Fop more liberty to gaze" (108). If indulging in "pretended fits" may advance the would-be wit and gentleman's claims to privilege and power, the coquette, Finch suggests, merely surrenders her freedom and subjectivity in exchange for the illusory power proffered by short-lived male solicitude. The poet diagnoses both fop and coquette as suffering from a "Defect in Sense" (110); this is the courtship behavior with which the "weaker Sort engage" (114). For Finch, the theatricality of courtship is a "pernicious Stage" (113), a preview of the trickery and mutual manipulation promised in the next act. Finch suggests that manipulation and discord must characterize marriage in a society that constructs women as passive objects, bereft of sexual and intellectual initiative.

Finch's ironic exploration of the role that the rhetoric of the spleen and hysteria play in domestic power struggles is likely informed by Sydenham's account of the challenge of soothing the hysteric:

They are very angry when any one speaks never so little of the hopes he has of their Recovery, easily believing that they undergo all the Miseries that can befall a man, foreboding the most dreadful things to themselves, entertaining their restless and anxious Breasts upon small occasions and perchance for none at all, Fear, Anger, Jealousie, Suspicion, and worse Passion of the Mind, if any can be worse, abhorring all Joy, Hope and Mirth.[29]

That Sydenham might be speaking in this passage as either husband or doctor is significant because the discourse of the spleen reinforces the custodial role of the husband while relegating every woman to the status of patient. If Finch holds the upper-class woman accountable for her participation in the theater of the spleen, she nevertheless suggests that the male actor enjoys a distinct advantage when any assertion of feminine autonomy can be easily reduced to mere hysteria. "Lordly *Man*" may be "born to Imperial Sway" (61), but a wife who demands any right is merely "Imperious" and hysterical. If the "Imperious" wife excuses her "o'erheated Passions" (54) under the cover of the "Vapours" and alternately "soften[s]" her husband's heart with "o'er-cast and show'ring Eyes" (57), whatever "disputed Point" is yielded, she is merely indulged as a child and an invalid. In the battle over some "contested Field" of power within the household (60), the husband "Compounds for Peace, to make that Right away" (62), surrendering a minor point in exchange for dismissing any acknowledgment of woman's autonomy, her just claim to "rights." At the same time, the spleen is the "sullen *Husband's* feign'd Excuse, / When the ill Humour with his Wife he spends, / and bears recruited Wit, and Spirits to his Friends" (91–93). The husband's wit is in fact recruited from the masculine ideology of the spleen and its medical patrons, who license the husband's "ill Humour" as a sign of wit and sophistication while they undermine the wife's struggle for autonomy as symptomatic of hysteria.

Finch's splenetic ode echoes and transforms Cowley's Pindaric "Upon Liberty" and, in so doing, suggests that the claim to masculine license and liberty is constructed on the containment and subjugation of woman. In "Upon Liberty" the Protean form of the Pindaric is depicted as the poetic embodiment of masculine freedom, the poet's liberation from the restraints of social conformity and implicitly from those imposed by a domestic existence:

> If Life should a well order'd Poem be . . .
> The more Heroique strain let others take,
>   Mine the Pindarique way I'l make:
> The Matter shall be grave, the Numbers loose and free,
> It shall not keep one setled pace of Time,
> In the same Tune it shall not always Chime. (III, 114–18)

Finch's lament that her own attempts at the Pindaric produce only "crampt Numbers" reflects her struggle against internalizing the public criticism that her commitment to her art elicits. If Finch would herself reject the "well-order'd" monotony of the upper-class wife and claim some measure of the artistic and social freedom that

Cowley claims for himself, she is well aware that her desires and ambitions will be read as signs of deviation from the social and natural order.[30]

Finch's ironic appropriation of the language of the spleen and of the form of the Pindaric nevertheless reflect her ongoing resistance to the specters of domestic containment and masculine devaluation by which she is haunted. The terminology of the spleen, Finch suggests, serves only to silence woman. In "The Introduction," as in "The Spleen," the narrow range of activities prescribed for woman by a patriarchal culture disabuses her of hopes for intellectual and artistic achievement and relegates her to a state of sociopolitical impotence and dependence:

> Alas! a woman that attempts the pen,
> Such an intruder on the rights of men . . .
> They tell us, we mistake our sex and way;
> Good breeding, fassion, dancing, dressing, play
> Are the accomplishments we shou'd desire;
> To write, or read, or think, or to enquire
> Wou'd cloud our beauty and exaust our time,
> And interrupt the Conquests of our prime;
> Whilst the dull mannage of a servile house
> Is held by some our utmost art, and use. (9,10, 13–20)

Finch anticipates the public censure that her own writing will elicit. Writing, for Finch and her contemporaries, is explicitly equated with challenging the political power of men. Its exclusion from the range of activities deemed "natural" to woman guarantees her silence and submission. The youthful "conquests" of the coquette provide only the fleeting satisfaction that precedes the literal servitude of the wife; the upper-class woman, whose household function is purely ornamental, is left in a state of debilitating self-absorption, preyed upon by the spleen.

In the explicit connections it invokes between the discourse of the spleen and the ideologies that justify women from medical certification, Elizabeth Tollet's "Hypatia," written in 1724, four years after Finch's death, echoes significant aspects of Finch's critique of the ideology of the spleen. The woman whose talents go undeveloped, whose "will" is "resigned to an imperious lord," is, as Tollet pronounces, "soured by spleen."[31] "Haughty man, unrivalled and alone, / May boast the world of science all his own," but his monopoly over the sciences can be maintained only by excluding women from education and training. He knows all too well, she suggests, that "ignorance will best obey."

The influence of Finch's critique is also echoed in Lady Wortley Montagu's little-known "Receipt to Cure the Vapours," published in 1748, twenty-four years after Finch's death, in which Lady Mary demystifies the attempts of the medical establishment to contain and neutralize women's sexuality. "I, like you, was born a woman," writes Montagu, addressing the Delia persona, "Well I know what vapours mean: / The disease, alas! is common; Single, we have all the spleen." She goes on to suggest that cures for the spleen justify the repression of women's desire: "All the morals that they tell us / Never cured the sorrow yet." If in prescribing marriage as a cure for her listener the speaker seems to argue for control, her euphemistic references to the benefits of heavy "doses" of daily conversation, or intercourse, constitute a poetic act of sexual transgression. Lady Mary reasserts the excesses of feminine desire; rather than the repression of desire, she prescribes its exhaustion. The ambiguity of the final stanza suggests also that the loss of the sexual desire that engenders "the spleen" may also come from playing the role of the passive wife who serves merely as an audience for her husband's thoughts. Both Tollet and Montagu appear to have understood Finch's "The Spleen" as reflecting on the resistance that is engendered by repression.

The "Proteus-like" spleen in Finch's account is identified not simply with masculinist discourses but with competing femininized narratives that it elicits, narratives that are identified in Finch's poem with the mystery and power of nature. "Whilst in the *Muses* Paths I stray," writes Finch, "My Hand delights to trace unusual Things / And deviates from the known, and common way." Finch's appropriation of the language of contingency and masculine privilege as a badge of the resistance of both woman and nature serves as an ironic commentary on masculinist science and poetry; though both the poet and the physician-experimentalist espouse voluntarist views and methodologies and proclaim their receptiveness to experience and the "otherness" of woman and nature, Finch suggests that the flexibility of Cowley's poetic form and Sydenham's diagnostic methodology serves only to advance the masculine freedom and license that is defined by the subjugation and exploitation of woman and feminized nature. The poem, in fact, offers an ironic critique of a stock rhetorical figure of the Royal Society that also appears in Sydenham. Though Sydenham's whiggish politics and insistence upon a radically inductive methodology distinguished him from Cowley, Harvey, and other members of the Royal Society and College of Physicians, Finch suggests that his gendering of hysteria and hypochondria participates in the coercive, masculinist ideology she critiques. The figure of feminized nature hounded by the male physician appears in a passage that serves as a bridge between Sydenham's discussion of his success in treating the smallpox and his remarks on hysteria and hypochondria. Sydenham touts the effectiveness of the contingent empiricism for which he was renowned and contrasts his own approach to the mere "Fictions" of classical medicine. The physician who is truly "Proficient in the Art of Physick" must "take so much Pains in the Art of Physick . . . in searching out that hidden and crooked method whereby Nature produces and nourishes Diseases." An approach that does any less "makes that which is called the Art of Physick, rather a babbling Faculty. . . . for the first Contrivers of Speculations had as great Contentions about their Brain-sick Fictions, as their Slaves and

Tools, and yet none of them perhaps in the right." Ironically, for Finch, the masculine ideology that Sydenham endorses is itself a "Brain-sick Fiction."[32]

Whatever political differences exist between Sydenham and Harvey, Finch suggests that they share crucial ideological suppositions of the sort evident in Cowley's ode to Harvey. The image of feminized nature at the mercy of the male experimentalist is prominent in Cowley's Ode "*Upon* Dr. Harvey," in which Harvey is depicted as tracking "Coy Nature" through the "winding streams of blood" until he corners her secret "retreat" in the inner sanctum of the heart:

> *Harvey* was with her there,
> And held this slippery *Proteus* in a chain,
> Till all her mighty Mysteries she descry'd,
> Which from his wit the attempt before to hide
> Was the first thing that Nature did in vain. (32–36)

Cowley depicts Harvey's insight into the circulation of the blood as a victory over a feminized nature that is raped and dominated. The poet goes on to sing the praises of the doctor, whose methods have provided an antidote to the diseased tradition of Galen:

> Great Doctor! Th'Art of Curing's cur'd by thee,
> We now thy patient Physick see,
> From all inveterate diseases free,
> Purg'd of old errors by thy care. (67–70)

Only in the closing lines of the poem does Cowley offer a perfunctory gesture of voluntarist humility, minimally conceding the doctor's mortality and admitting that "Nature now, so long by him surpass't, / Will sure have her revenge on him at last"(90–91). Finch appropriates the lines for her own voluntarist narrative to suggest that the misogynist constructions of nature and woman embodied in the discourse of the spleen and hysteria and in the patriarchal ideologies of Cowley, Harvey, and Sydenham are themselves "Brain-sick" fictions.

In her poem, the flexibility of the discourse of the spleen becomes a function of the resistance of both woman and nature to the strategies of patriarchal control and exploitation:

> Tho' the Physicians greatest Gains,
> Altho' his growing Wealth he sees
> Daily increas'd by Ladies Fees,
> Yet dost thou baffle all his studious Pains:
> Not skilful *Lower*, thy Sorce cou'd find,
> Or, thro the well-dissected Body trace
> The secret, the mysterious ways,
> By which thou dost surprize, and prey upon the Mind
> Tho' in the Search, too deep for Humane Thought,
> With unsuccessful Toil he wrought,
> 'Till, thinking Thee to've catch'd, Himself by thee was caught,
> Retain'd thy Pris'ner, thy acknowledg'd Slave,
> And sunk beneath thy Chain to a lamented Grave. (138–50)

In invoking the suicide of Richard Lower, who was a protégé of Harvey and Willis, Finch implicitly implicates Harvey, Willis, and the other physician-virtuosi of the Royal College of Physicians and Royal Society in the kind of self-defeating and inconsistent behavior that they displace onto their female patients. Following the death of Willis, Lower, a member of the Royal Society and of the Royal College of Physicians was recognized as perhaps the most preeminent physician in London until he fell from political and social favor for his support for the Titus Oates Plot of 1678. Oates and his co-conspirators inflamed anti-Catholic Whig sentiments by fabricating stories of a plotted coup to place James, then duke of York, on the throne. As a loyal follower of James, Finch implicitly invokes Lower's participation in the plot, equating it with the moral weakness and instability that the discourse of the spleen implicitly essentializes as feminine.

The passage may, moreover, be read as an allusion to Lower's—and implicitly Harvey's—well-known enthusiasm for vivisection and dissection, linking animal experimentation with the violence that the male physician/virtuoso perpetrates upon women's bodies in the name of medicine.[33] In Finch's poem the physician-experimentalists' quest for the underlying causes of "the spleen" is associated with violence against both nature and the bodies of women patients. Finch implies that the medical terminology that fosters a view of woman as inherently pathological reflects man's frustrated attempt to at once dominate and root out the source of his own desire. This frustration, she suggests, is enacted in violence against the bodies of women, which, though "well," are nevertheless symbolically and literally dismembered by physician-experimentalists. In Finch's voluntarist narrative, the "secret and mysterious ways" of God, which the members of the Royal Society would preserve, are displaced by a sublime principle that resists all definition, fusing the masculine and the feminine and eliciting masculine fear in the process.

Finch's ostensibly innocuous reference to the "threatning Angel and the speaking Ass"(89) strikes at the heart of the masculine anxiety that underlies the discourse of the spleen, and more generally, the conventional construction of feminine virtue and corruption. The tableau of the "threatning Angel and the speaking Ass," depicting the biblical tale of the prophet Balaam and his donkey, was one of several images—including that of the face of the monarch—that, according to Katherine Rogers, splenetic ladies embroidered on silk or painted on glass by orders of the medical establishment.[34] Finch registers her resistance to regimens that are designed to occupy women with traditional domestic tasks and neutralize any threat they might pose to masculine autonomy, asserting that she will not

> in fading Silks compose
>> Faintly th'inimitable *Rose*,
> Fill up an ill-drawn *Bird,* or paint on glass
> The *Sov'reign's* blurr'd and undistinguish'd Face,
> The Threatning *Angel* and the speaking *Ass.* (85–89)

McGovern suggests that Finch's reference to the reduction of the sovereign's face to a "blurred and undistinguish'd" image and the tableau of the "threatning Angel and the speaking Ass" are both emblematic of the poet's resistance to the reign of William of Orange.³⁵ The tableau, I believe, also reflects on the genealogy and method of Finch's poetry of resistance. In the biblical tale, Balaam, who rides out to battle with the Israelites, beats his donkey—gendered as female—for refusing to advance down a road blocked by an angel visible only to the donkey and sent by God to kill the prophet. Balaam continues to beat the animal until the donkey speaks, demanding to know why she is beaten, whereupon the angel intervenes. The angel repeats the donkey's complaints, castigating Balaam for beating her. He informs Balaam that if he had continued in his path the angel would have killed him but spared the donkey's life. While the beating of the ass is undoubtedly suggestive of the oppression that Finch associates with the rule of William of Orange, one also has to take into account the gendering of the ass as female. In this respect, the tableau may be seen as offering a vivid image of the physical and emotional violence against women of the upper classes that is authorized by the male physician and experimentalist. With its insistence upon locating the source of the spleen within woman herself, the terminology of the disease mystifies the results of repression and abuse. Finch, then, licenses her own struggles against patriarchal tyranny by associating her oppression with the violence enacted against James II. The monarchy remains, for Finch, the model for her own sovereign subjectivity.[36]

For Finch, though the construction of woman as passive angel, delicate as the fine embroidery that so absorbs her attention, strips her of her suspect sexuality, she nevertheless continues to be viewed with suspicion. At any moment she might, like Finch, assert her autonomy, lay claim to the authority of the patriarch, displace or conflate divine speech with her own. The construction of woman as angel, therefore, both mystifies and facilitates the reduction of woman to "speaking Ass," a bestial and servile figure whose speech is, by definition, chaotic. The chaotic speech of the ass suggests the elliptical speech of the hysteric, who, like Freud's Dora, refuses to be reduced, who insists on authoring her own narrative, on the subjective and political order in ostensible disorder.[38] If other women drew some satisfaction from futile acts of resistance against the repressiveness of patriarchal authority by reducing the face of the monarch to a "blurred and undistinguished" image, Finch represents herself as engaging in a more public and vocal form of resistance.[39] Finch's poetry emerges out of and is elicited by repression. The tableau of the "threatning Angel and the speaking Ass," like Finch's ostensibly innocuous allusion to it, embodies the possibility for subversion that lies in claiming the language of the oppressor and using it to demystify and subvert the goals it has served. In Finch's own resistant poetics, the categories of subject and object, of hysteria and reason, of "science" and literature, of ass, prophet, and angel collapse. The spleen itself becomes the topic, source, and substance of Finch's art; it is transformed through the poem into a cure for the medical establishment that would prescribe for woman the limits of her artistic and intellectual capabilities. If Finch finds within a masculine poetic tradition a form loose enough to serve her, as a woman writer, she nevertheless defies the standards of eighteenth-century social and poetic order. Finch's poem transforms "the spleen" into a site of contested meaning, offering an anatomy of

the semiotic systems by which disease is signified and a broader
critique of the cultural and political underpinnings of scientific dis-
course. The masculinist discourses of Restoration natural philosophy,
medicine, and poetry, in Finch's account, become indistinguishable
from the feminized mutability they would describe and contain;
they are, as Sydenham described the hysteric, "constant only to
Inconstancy."[40] The representatives of patriarchal control are them-
selves, moreover, ultimately reduced in Finch's poem into a single
"blurr'd and undistinguish'd Face" that serves also as a disturbing
reminder of the poet's complex and conflicted relationship to the
authority of a monarch, whose power had so longer authorized her
own privileged place at court.

AFTERWORD

An Anatomy of the Handmaid's Tale

I stumbled upon Boyle's reference to natural philosophy as the "Handmaid to Divinity" quite late in my research. Pondering the implications of Boyle's unconscious pun has taken my study in directions that I could not have predicted, impelling me toward a more coherent formulation of the relationships among theology, gender, and natural philosophy as it was theorized and practiced under the auspices of both church and state in seventeenth-century England. Donna Haraway has referred to the Western scientist's claim to the encompassing and disembodied "god trick of seeing everywhere from nowhere." Through my readings of the poems of Donne and Milton, in particular, I have sought to elucidate the roots of the "god trick" in theology. As a supplement to Scripture and theology, as a "Handmaid to Divinity," the "new philosophies" served a critical role in legitimating the authority of monarchy, and patriarchy, and in impelling—and indeed sanctifying—the techno-logical transformation of the natural world into an emblem of the power of God—and of godly English gentlemen.

Haraway has offered the figure of the Coyote or Trickster in the narratives of Indians of the American Southwest as a starting point for envisioning responsible and responsive scientific theories and practices that recognize and respect the agency of a natural world that will continually "hoodwink" us, resisting our best efforts to know it, as it resists all strategies for mastering it.[1] In various ways, and to vary-ing degrees, the poetry of Donne, Milton, and Finch resonates with the figure of the Trickster. For Donne and Milton in particular, God is a trickster, an accomplice in the Coyote games of nature, in undermining strategies for advancing monarchical power and, in Milton's case, the power and privileges of a landed elite. In this sense, the poetry of Donne and Milton demonstrates the limitations of accounts by both literary critics and historians that assume that theological challenges to the emergent discourses of Western science are necessarily reactionary. The limitations of these accounts mark a broader failure within the academy to acknowledge the insights of scholars such as Christopher Hill, Nigel Smith, and Phyllis Mack, who have explored the role that radical readings of Scripture have played in undermining the hierarchies of class and gender in seventeenth-century England.[2] There are, moreover, numerous other examples that one can cite of the effective deployment of theological claims in the service of progressive or radical politics. In the last few decades, liberation theology has played an important role in struggles for land reform in Latin America. In the United States, religion helped to mobilize both the nineteenth-century abolitionist movement and the Civil Rights movement. More recently, inner-city churches in particular have actively spearheaded and supported many of the organizing efforts that collectively compose the environmental justice movement.

My readings of all three poets suggest that seventeenth-century poetry may serve as a valuable resource in the emergent field of ecotheology, a field that is engaged in contesting theological claims and scriptural readings that justify the exploitation and domination of nature. The *Anniversaries*, book 8 of *Paradise Lost*, and "The Spleen" all demonstrate, to varying degrees, that the exploitation of nature and the exploitation of humans are intimately interrelated. Like the contemporary environmental justice movement, the concerns that book 8 of *Paradise Lost* raises about the interrelationship between the exploitation of nature and the exploitation of workers, in particular, provide a mandate for scrutinizing and developing the intersections between ecotheology and liberation theology.

Finch, more than either Donne or Milton, recognizes the material implications of the misogynist discourses and assumptions of virtuoso and experimental physician as they impinge upon her own life. She is an early instance of a lengthy tradition of women writers whose work challenges the ideologies of Western science. Finch recognizes that her own rights and the rights of nature are closely connected, linked by the metaphors and gendered ideologies that will inform, for centuries, the claims and practices of research scientists and medical practitioners. Finch's poem anticipates developments that future women writers such as Margaret Atwood will explore in more explicit and disturbing detail. In the theocratic and rigidly stratified world of Atwood's novel *The Handmaid's Tale*, physicians play a central role in policing the sexuality of women, whose sole value lies in their reproductive function, a function that ensures the continuity of a small patriarchal elite. Unlike the handmaid of Atwood's tale, however, Finch, as a former maid of honor to Mary of Modena, remains, like Donne, fundamentally disengaged from the concerns of the lower classes, of women and men whose laboring bodies are the "natural" resources upon which her own privileged life depends. The critiques that she, Donne, and Milton offer demonstrate the limitations of their own partial and situated vision as this study does my own.

While Haraway warns against the futility of the "search for the fetishized perfect subject of oppositional history," the metaphor of the handmaid nonetheless serves as a disturbing reminder of the limitations of my own study, and of the need for more complete accounts of the effect of science on the laboring class in England and on the inhabitants of the New/Old Worlds. This area of study seems particularly urgent in light of the concerns raised by the environmental justice movement in recent years. If science can, as Bacon insisted, serve as an instrument for "the relief of man's estate," historically that relief has been distributed extremely unevenly.[3] While the poor, Native Americans, and people of color in general have little access to health care and generally receive comparatively few of the material benefits of techno-science, they suffer disproportionately from the toxic by-products of industry and technology.

The skeptical reevaluations that Milton and Finch offer of the roles that a contingent method and rhetoric play in advancing the claims of the Royal Society are particularly relevant today in light of the strategies that corporations routinely adopt to forestall regulatory legislation. As Robert Proctor and others have observed, corporations increasingly invoke the contingency of scientific claims and practices to justify the endless proliferation of scientific studies, thus enabling them to maximize profits and evade accountability.[4] The poems of Milton and Finch demonstrate the effective limits of the commitment to narrative revolution that Donne deploys strategically in the *Anniversaries* to enshrine his own poetic authority and contest the authority of natural philosophers and astronomers who would advance Jacobean absolutism. At present, the contemporary fetishization of contingency within the academy not only runs the risk of invalidating the universal and metaphysical claims that have undergirded countless popular resistance movements but also obscures the extent to which contingent methods and rhetorics can be deployed to justify reactionary political agendas. The quest for a perfectly contingent and nonessentializing rhetoric and theory that continues to occupy so much of contemporary academic discourse reinscribes the assumptions and values of the language projection schemes of the seventeenth century in its unshaken belief that the central conflicts of our time—conflicts rooted in real, material inequities—are subject to discursive resolution within the academy. In calling into question the variable uses of a contingent method and rhetoric, the poems of Donne, Milton, and Finch suggest that we would do well to concern ourselves less with whether knowledge claims are *framed* as totalizing or contingent and devote greater attention to scrutinizing the specific material and ideological interests that are identified with, and served by, those claims, and to considering the claims and interests of those who continue to be excluded from participation in the ostensibly "consensual" production of knowledge claims.

In the last few years, in developing undergraduate coursework in ecological issues in American literature, I have found myself reading about cancer clusters, about dropping sperm counts and rising rates of miscarriages, birth defects, and autoimmune disorders. I followed the progress of numerous friends in various stages of treatment and recovery from cancer, listening while a thirty-three-year-old colleague pondered a preventive mastectomy on learning that her thirty-four-year-old sister had been diagnosed with a malignancy. Two years ago I was diagnosed with a melanoma, which I was lucky enough to detect in its very early stages. Every day this past winter, as I drove home from campus, trucks stacked with some of the last ancient forest in the Pacific Northwest passed me on the Interstate, and every evening I read stories in the *Oregonian* about protesters camped out in the pouring rain to block the logging trucks. In working on this manuscript, I have come to question many of the hypotheses with which I began, discarding many of the beliefs I originally held about the differences between literature and science. In working on the dialogue on astronomy in particular, I was reminded of the need to challenge ourselves repeatedly to ensure that research in the humanities is not an evasion of the material concerns and struggles of the Garden, but a contribution, albeit small, to those struggles. For now, I hold out the perhaps naive hope that seventeenth-century poetry will have some material role in fostering a skepticism that will encourage readers to question and challenge the claims of corporate-sponsored and corporate-influenced studies that call all in doubt for the express purpose of mystifying the material effects of techno-science on the ecosystem and on the minds and bodies of those of us who depend upon it.

NOTES

Introduction

1. See Latour and Woolgar, *Laboratory Life;* Biagioli, *Galileo, Courtier;* Biagioli, "Galileo the Emblem Maker"; Biagioli, "Galileo's System of Patronage"; Merchant, *The Death of Nature;* Haraway, *Simians, Cyborgs, and Women;* Rouse, *Knowledge and Power;* Rouse, "What Are Cultural Studies of Scientific Knowledge?"; Londa Schiebinger, *The Mind Has No Sex?;* Shapin and Schaffer, *Leviathan and the Air-Pump;* and Shapin, *A Social History of Truth.*

2. See Knoespel, "The Emplotment of Chaos: Instability and Narrative Order."

3. See Toulmin, "The Construal of Reality: Criticism in Modern and Postmodern Science."

4. On the contributions of both Hueper and Carson to an understanding of the environmental health crisis, see Proctor, *Cancer Wars,* esp. 35–54; see also Carson, *Silent Spring;* on Theodora Colborn and research on endocrine disruptors, see Colborn, Dumanoski, and Myers, *Our Stolen Future.*

5. On the environmental justice movement, see Bullard, ed., *Unequal Protection;* Bullard, *Dumping in Dixie;* Hurley, *Environmental Inequalities;* Hofrichter, ed., *Toxic Struggles;* Gottlieb, *Forcing the Spring;* Bryant and Mohai, eds., *Race and the Incidence of Environmental Hazards.*

6. See Batt, *Patient No More,* esp. 213–58.

7. World Health Organization, *The Prevention of Cancer,* 4.

8. Rogers, *The Matter of Revolution.*

9. See Martin, *Francis Bacon, the State and the Reform of Natural Philosophy.* See also Robert Stillman's treatment of Bacon in *The New Philosophy and Universal Languages in Seventeenth-Century England.*

10. See Hill, *The World Turned Upside Down*, and *The Collected Essays of Christopher Hill*, vol. 2.

11. Hill, *Collected Essays*, 83.

12. See Markley, "Objectivity as Ideology," "Representing Order," and *Fallen Languages*. On the complex relationship between Protestant theology and science, see also Easlea, *Witch Hunting, Magic and the New Philosophy*; Markley, "Robert Boyle on Language"; Jacob, *Robert Boyle and the English Revolution*, "Restoration Ideologies and the Royal Society," and "Restoration, Reformation, and the Origins of the Royal Society"; Burtt, *The Metaphysical Foundations of Modern Science*; and Westfall, *Science and Religion in Seventeenth-Century England*.

13. Keller, *Reflections on Gender and Science*, 33–43. See Mark Breitenberg's *Anxious Masculinity in Early Modern England*, esp. 69–97. Merrens, "Exchanging Cultural Capital," examines the links between Bacon's rhetoric of domination over feminized nature and the "strategies for gendering and manipulating power" in *Astrophil and Stella*. For a consideration of the relationship between science, colonialism, and gender, see also Albanese, *New Science, New World*.

14. See Shapin and Schaffer, *Leviathan*.

15. Shapin and Schaffer, *Leviathan*, 78.

16. Latour and Woolgar, *Laboratory Life*, 46.

17. See Latour and Woolgar, *Laboratory Life*, esp. 43–88 and 189–230.

18. Boyle, *The Excellency of Theology, as Compar'd with Natural Philosophy*, 158.

19. Sidney, *An Apologie for Poetrie*, 8.

20. Stillman, *The New Philosophy*, 95.

21. Donne, *Second Anniversary*, ll. 326, 328, 329–30, in *The Variorum Edition of the Poetry of John Donne*.

22. Shapin and Schaffer, *Leviathan*, 65.

23. For studies on the rhetoric of probability and certainty, contingency and closure, see Hacking, *The Emergence of Probability*; Shapiro, *Probability and Certainty in Seventeenth-Century England*; and Kroll, *The Material Word*, 49–79. While Kroll assumes that the rhetoric of probability and contingency displaces the rhetoric of certainty and closure in the Restoration, Stillman's *The New Philosophy* provides a more nuanced discussion of the relationship between contingent and totalizing claims and explores more fully the coercive uses of the rhetoric of contingency.

24. On the displacement of women from women's health care in the seventeenth and eighteenth centuries, see Landry and McLean, "Of Forceps, Patents, and Paternity"; and Schiebinger, *The Mind Has No Sex?*, esp. 102–18 and 189–213.

25. See Laqueur, *Making Sex*. Stepan, "Race and Gender," demonstrates that the metaphorical matrices that linked the cranial weights and structures of women, blacks, and apes in late eighteenth- and nineteenth-century medical representations served to perpetuate the place of white males atop the hierarchies of gender and race. Gould, The *Mismeasure of Man*, explores the use of analogies linking the cranial weights and structures of blacks and women to those of apes in the nineteenth century.

26. See Cixous, "Sorties"; Clement,"The Guilty One"; and Gilbert and Gubar, *The Madwoman in the Attic*. On the social construction of madness, see Foucault, *Madness and Civilization*.

27. See Salvaggio, *Enlightened Absence*, esp. 9–11.

28. Serres, *Hermes*, xiii.

29. Salvaggio, *Enlightened Absence*, 9–11.

30. Haraway, *Simians, Cyborgs, and Women*, 195.

Chapter 1. Francis Bacon and the Advancement of Absolutism

1. See, for example, Marotti, *John Donne, Coterie Poet*, 235–45. Though Marotti's reading provides essential insights that inform my own exploration of the poems, it does not acknowledge the extent to which the poet implicates natural philosophy and astronomy in his critique of the patronage economy and of the corruptions of the Jacobean court. In a much earlier study, "Religious Cynicism in Donne's Poetry," Marius Bewley argued that the poems reflect Donne's cynicism about both religion and patronage. Annabel Patterson's "John Donne, Kingsman?" provides important new insights into the *Anniversaries* as they critique the king's prerogative. She does not, however, address connections to the New Philosophy. The most in-depth study of natural philosophy and astronomy in the *Anniversaries* remains Charles Coffin's *John Donne and the New Philosophy*. Coffin treats "science" as objective, progressive, and apolitical and sees Donne as responding to an emergent split between science and theology by embracing a skeptical fideism. While Marjorie Hope Nicolson, invoking R. G. Collingwood, notes the analogical basis of all knowledge claims, she does not see evidence of Donne and his contemporaries as possessing this insight; she also does not address the ideological implications of the analogies that shape science (see *The Breaking of the Circle*). In the most recent in-depth study of the poems, *Donne's Idea of a Woman*, Tayler argues that the central conceit of the

poems reflects Donne's commitment to a scholastic epistemology. Tayler does not attempt to examine the broader ideological implications of this ostensible commitment.

2. Martin, *Francis Bacon*, 102.

3. Donne, *The Courtier's Library*, 43–44.

4. Cited in Carey, *John Donne*, 17.

5. Ibid.

6. Ibid., 66.

7. Bald, *John Donne*, 93–94.

8. In "Religious Cynicism in Donne's Poetry," Bewley described the poems as a "deliberate dramatization of the unsavory aspects of Donne's situation, a cryptic indictment of the motives Donne had gradually been compelled to act on in his search for worldly advancement" (633). On Donne and the politics of patronage, see Carey, *John Donne*, 60–130; Marotti, *John Donne*, esp. 152–274; Marotti, "John Donne and the Rewards of Patronage"; and Dubrow, "Sun in Water."

9. Donne, *Courtier's Library*, 51, 73.

10. Marwil, *Trials of Counsel*, 80.

11. In her introduction to *The Courtier's Library*, Evelyn M. Simpson observes that "There is nothing in these items of the personal bitterness which envenoms Donne's attack on Bacon, the false friend of Essex" (23).

12. Bald, *John Donne*, 113.

13. Bald, *Donne and the Drurys*, 38, 30.

14. Judson, *Crisis of the Constitution*, 20, 23, 82.

15. Ibid., 142.

16. For a summary of the tradition of the common law and Bacon's proposals for its reform, see Martin, *Francis Bacon*, 72–139. See also Levack, "Law and Ideology," and Helgerson, *Forms of Nationhood*, 65–110.

17. Hawarde, *Les Reportes del Cases in Camera Stellata*, 188, cited in Knafla; Knafla, *Law and Politics in Jacobean England*, 176, 76, 148, 89.

18. Spedding, *The Letters and the Life of Francis Bacon* 6:38, 3:371.

19. Judson, *Crisis of the Constitution*, 153.

20. Ibid., 133.

21. Cobbett, *Complete Collection of State Trials* 2:581, 595.

22. Judson, *Crisis of the Constitution*, 165, 143.

23. Walton initiated a critical tradition, which received strong reinforcement from Edmund Gosse and Bald, of viewing the author of *Pseudo-Martyr* as an

unambiguous defender of royal authority. John Carey sees Donne as fully embracing James's absolutist ideology in order to advance his career. A number of studies in recent years have complicated this portrait of Donne, identifying subversive challenges to the prerogative in both *Pseudo-Martyr* and *Biathanatos*, as well as in the sermons. See, for example, Shami, "Kings and Desperate Men"; Patterson, "John Donne, Kingsman?"; Patterson, "All Donne"; Norbrook, "The Monarch of Wit and the Republic of Letters"; and Harland, "Donne's Political Intervention in the Parliament of 1629." *Biathanatos* was written in 1607 or 1608.

24. See Strier's insightful analysis in "Radical Donne."

25. At the same time, Donne problematizes the relationship between nature and culture, pointing to the historical and cultural contingency of, for example, St. Paul's assertion that long hair was an indication of "'delicacy and effeminateness'" (Marotti, *John Donne*, 190). While Strier sees *Biathanatos* as resting sovereign authority in the individual conscience, he reads *Pseudo-Martyr* as demonstrating a more conservative ideology.

26. Donne, *Biathanatos*, 127; Marotti, *John Donne*, 190; Patterson, "John Donne, Kingsman?" 257.

27. Ibid., 260–61; Patterson, "All Donne," 37–38. On Donne's participation in the Mermaid Club, see also Shapiro, "The Mermaid Club."

28. Donne, *Pseudo-Martyr*, n. p., 43–44.

29. *Courtier's Library*, 50–51; Gleason, "Dr. Donne in the Court of Kings."

30. Biagioli, "Galileo the Emblem Maker," 230, 232. See also Biagioli, *Galileo, Courtier*, 1–10.

31. Bacon, *Works* 3:263.

32. Galileo, *Siderius nuncius*, 29, 30.

33. Biagioli, *Galileo, Courtier*, 53; Galileo, *Sidereus nuncius*, 31.

34. Bacon, *Letters* 6:90–91.

35. Bacon, *Works* 3:348; see especially Martin, *Francis Bacon*, 141–71. My argument builds on Martin's to explore more fully the role that Bacon's natural philosophy would play in buttressing the theological basis of an expanded prerogative. See also Stillman, *New Philosophy*, 55–112, on Bacon and Jacobean absolutism.

36. Bacon, *Works* 3:222. For an overview of views of Adamic language in the period, see Bono, *Word of God*, esp. 48–84, 216; see Bono's critique of Whitney's conception of Bacon's ostensibly "metaleptic stance" (221–26).

37. Bacon, *Works* 3:396.

38. Ibid. 3:388–89.

39. See Bono, *Word of God*, 216–19; Bacon, *Works* 3:350.

40. Ibid. 3:300–301.

41. Ibid. 3:298–99.

42. Ibid. 3:299.

43. Ibid. 3:267, 268.

44. Stillman, *New Philosophy*, 107, 104. Whitney observes in *Francis Bacon and Modernity* that "the difference between the analogical and inductive processes remains partly just a question of quantity and meticulousness: more data, properly sifted, will yield better generalizations" (79); he overlooks, however, the importance of prosthetic technologies as a distinctive feature of Bacon's inductive method. Bacon, *Works* 3:370. See Julie Solomon's insightful article, "To Know, to Fly, to Conjure," in which she examines Bacon's "intentional effacing of self and its immediate interests" in relationship to the discursive practices of merchants and travelers in the period. Solomon's book *Objectivity in the Making* was published too recently to be addressed in this study.

45. Stillman, *The New Philosophy*, 105–8; Bacon, *Works* 3:394. Bacon variously entertains notions of a "real character" and of hieroglyphics as the means for communicating the "true" nature of things disclosed by the natural philosopher. On Bacon's interest in hieroglyphics, see also Elsky, *Authorizing Words*, 147–84. Bacon's views of hieroglyphics, as Elsky notes, departs from existing conceptions in the Renaissance. For Bacon hieroglyphs are "pictures of the thing (or idea) to which they refer. . . . Unlike the highly symbolic hieroglyph of Renaissance tradition, Bacon's hieroglyph is univocal, rather than opaque, and it has a clear and singular rather than an engimatic relationship to its meaning" (175). See also Bono, *Word of God*, 176–78, 237–39.

46. Jardine, *Francis Bacon*, 115.

47. On the oppositional relationship that Bacon constructs between poetic idealization and scientific realism, see Schuler, *Francis Bacon;* see also Dollimore, *Radical Tragedy*, esp. 75–80.

48. Bacon, *The Wisedome of the Ancients*, n. p.; Puttenham, *The Arte of English Poesie*, 9; Sidney, *An Apologie for Poetrie*, 38.

49. Patterson, *Censorship and Interpretation*, 29; Puttenham, *Arte of English Poesie*, 38.

50. Bacon, *Essays*, 124–25; Patterson, *Censorship and Interpretation*, 14.

51. Bacon, *Works* 3:343.

52. Bacon, *Wisedome of the Ancients*, n.p.

53. Ibid.

54. Ibid., 22, 37–38.

55. Ibid., 22, 35.

56. Ibid., 37; Whitney, *Francis Bacon*, 161.

57. See Merchant, *The Death of Nature*, esp. 164–90.

58. Bacon, *Works* 4:253.

59. Bacon, *The Wisedome of the Ancients*, 69–70.

60. See Merchant's discussion of women, witchcraft and nature (*Death of Nature*, 127–63), and her discussion of Bacon's rhetoric of torture (168–72).

61. See Foucault, *Discipline and Punish*.

62. Cormack, "Twisting the Lion's Tail," 78.

63. Hunt, "Spectral Origins of the English Revolution," 310–11; see Nicolson, *Breaking of the Circle*, 91–96; see also Haydn, *The Counter-Renaissance*; Yates, *Astraea*, 54, 11.

64. See Parry, *The Golden Age Restor'd*, 72–74.

65. Cormack, "Twisting the Lion's Tale," 70, 66, 28.

66. Parry, *Golden Age Restor'd*, 82–83.

67. Jill Peláez Baumgaertner sees Donne as at once "lavishly memorializ[ing] the dead child, and compliment[ing] the Prince of Wales" ("Political Play and Theological Uncertainty in the *Anniversaries*," 46).

68. Hunt, "Spectral Origins," 312.

69. Donne, "Elegie on the Untimely Death of the Incomparable Prince, Henry," *Complete English Poems*, 288–91.

70. Donne, *Sermons* 3:227.

71. Ibid., 229–30.

72. Ibid., 230.

73. Augustine observes: "Have we spoken or announced anything worthy of God? Rather I feel that I have done nothing but wish to speak: If I have spoken, I have not said what I wished to say. Whence do I know this, except because God is ineffable? . . . For God, although nothing worthy may be spoken of Him, has accepted the tribute of the human voice and wished to take joy in praising Him with out words" (*On Christian Doctrine*, 10–11).

74. Donne, *Sermons* 3:171.

75. Ibid. 3:225–26.

76. Donne, *Essays in Divinity*, 49.

77. See Guibbory, "Oh, let mee not serve so."

78. Smith, *Donne: Songs and Sonets*, 8; Docherty, *John Donne Undone*, 62.

79. Dubrow, *Echoes of Desire*, 203–48; Estrin, *Laura*, 181; see also Kerrigan, "What Was Donne Doing?"; Benet, "Sexual Transgression in Donne's Elegies," 15; see Guibbory, "Oh, let mee not serve so" and "Donne, Milton and Holy Sex."

80. Donne, *Complete English Poems*, 48–50, 126–28, 18.

81. Ibid., 36–37, 8–9.

Chapter 2. John Donne's *Anniversaries*

1. Aers and Kress, "Dark Texts Need Notes"; Marotti, *John Donne, Coterie Poet*, esp. 203–32; Dubrow, "Sun in Water" and *Echoes of Desire*, esp. 210–48.

2. While he has suggested that Jonson's comment may have been intended to elicit an explanation from Donne, John Carey believes that Donne's response should be taken at face value. He suggests that Donne was "trying to stretch language to make it embody the most exaggerated things that could be thought. It was a voyage into the undiscovered spaces of hyperbole" (*John Donne*, 103). Arguing that Donne represents Drury as a regenerate soul in whom the image of the divine is restored, Barbara Lewalski positions the poems within the generic boundaries of classical and Renaissance epideictic poetry; see *Donne's "Anniversaries" and the Poetry of Praise*, esp. 42–70.

3. Mueller, "Women among the Metaphysicals."

4. Marotti, *Coterie Poet*, 203, 207.

5. Hall, "To the Praise of the Dead and the Anatomy," in *The Variorum Edition of the Poetry of John Donne*, 5; subsequent references are to this edition and are identified by lone citations in the text.

6. Biagioli, *Galileo, Courtier*, 5.

7. Donne, *Essays in Divinity*, 40–41.

8. In "Religious Cynicism in Donne's Poetry," Marius Bewley, as I will note, associates "she" with the Catholic Church; Frank Manley identifies her with the Shekinah figured in the writings of Christian cabbalists in *John Donne: "The Anniversaries"* (Baltimore: Johns Hopkins UP, 1964); William Empson sees Donne's "she" as representing the Logos in *English Pastoral Poetry* (New York: Norton, 1938); Richard E. Hughes associates "she" with a variety of figures, including Dante's Beatrice, in "The Woman in Donne's *Anniversaries*," *ELH* 34 (1967): 307–26; Louis Martz sees Elizabeth Drury figured forth in the poems as the "symbol of a virtuous soul" in *The Poetry of Meditation* (New Haven, Conn.: Yale UP, 1954), 211–48; and most recently, in "Political Play and Theological

Uncertainty in the *Anniversaries*," Jill Peláez Baumgaertner sees Donne's "she" as conflating Drury and Prince Henry.

9. Nicolson, *Breaking of the Circle*, 79.

10. In the most recent study on the *Anniversaries*, however, Baumgaertner discusses Astraea in connection with the political iconography of Prince Henry but does not scrutinize this iconography in relationship to Henry's imperialist ambitions; she sees the poems as conflating Drury and Henry to offer praise to the Prince. See "Political Play and Theological Uncertainty in the *Anniversaries*."

11. Bewley, "Religious Cynicism."

12. Bacon, *Wisedom of the Ancients*, 19.

13. Dubrow, *Echoes of Desire*, 215.

14. Ibid., 11.

15. Ibid., 91.

16. Donne, *First Anniversary*, ll. 67–78, in *The Variorum Edition of the Poetry of John Donne*; subsequent references to the *Anniversaries* are to this edition and are identified by line citations in the text with the abbreviations FA and SA for *First Anniversary* and *Second Anniversary* respectively.

17. I am indebted to Simon Schaffer for this insight.

18. Montaigne, *Essayes*, 471–72.

19. Mayr, *Authority, Liberty, and Automatic Machinery in Early Modern Europe*, 124.

20. Montaigne, *Essayes*, 396.

21. Bacon, *Works* 3:364, 406.

22. Ibid. 3:292, 293.

23. Ibid. 3:293.

24. Ibid. 3:395.

25. Bacon, *Works* 3:389.

26. Montaigne, *Essayes*, 543–44.

27. See Martin, *Francis Bacon*, 164–71.

28. The reference to the "embarr'd" "commerce between heaven and earth" might be read as drawing a connection between Bacon's role in granting monopolies, and his attempts to assert a monopoly on divine truth through his natural philosophy.

29. Bacon, *Works* 3:370.

30. Adams, "One Direction for Donne's Skepticism," 84.

31. Bacon, *Letters* 3:26.

Chapter 3. The Fall of Science in Book 8 of *Paradise Lost*

1. See Webster, *The Great Instauration*, 1–31.

2. Milton, *Complete Poems and Major Prose*, 606.

3. On Milton's relationship to the Hartlib circle, see Lewalski, "Milton and the Hartlib Circle."

4. John Rogers's study *The Matter of Revolution*, which I discuss later in this chapter, provides important new insights into the ideological implications of Milton's vitalist beliefs. Though Rogers acknowledges the ideological reverberations in the dialogue on astronomy, he defers to John Guillory's reading of the dialogue in "From the Superfluous to the Supernumerary." Guillory's reading of the relationship between gender, astronomy, and the material economy of the garden in book 8 differs substantially from my own. My reading of Milton's response as a specific critique of the coercive ideologies he associates with astronomy and natural philosophy in Restoration England also differs markedly from Denise Albanese's reading of astronomy in *Paradise Lost* in *New Science, New World*. Albanese makes the problematic assertion that while Milton seeks to "demonize" (143) the emergent discourses and technologies of early modern science, they nevertheless repeatedly erupt into the text, thereby undermining Milton's attempts to rehabilitate an embattled and, in Albanese's account, undifferentiated Christian humanism. While Albanese's study offers a number of important insights, it oversimplifies the complex relationship between theology and natural philosophy and astronomy and represents these emergent discourses as constituting an unproblematic epistemic break between "universalizing theology and contingent history" (126). Amy Boesky's "Milton, Galileo, and Sunspots" sees the poet as skeptical of the prosthetic capabilities of optics and, in particular, of their coercive uses in facilitating colonialist expansion. While it devotes little attention to the dialogue on astronomy, Stanley Fish's *Surprized by Sin* remains one of the most insightful examinations of Milton's attitude toward natural philosophy in the period; see, in particular, 107–30. Christopher Hill's *Milton and the English Revolution* does not deal with the issue in depth, but Hill does acknowledge that the "victory of experimental science" reflects and reinforces the defeat of Milton's republican ideals (401). Treatments of the dialogue on astronomy by Jacobus, *Sudden Apprehension*; Lovejoy, "Milton's Dialogue on Astronomy"; Nicolson, *Science and Imagination*, 80–109; Nicolson, *John Milton*, 271–73; Svendsen, *Milton and Science*; and most recently, Marjara, *Contemplation of Created Things*, have largely overlooked the political concerns that it reflects.

5. McColley, "Milton's Dialogue on Astronomy."

6. See Fowler's edition of *Paradise Lost*, 402n.

7. Nicolson, *Breaking of the Circle*, 184. If, as Guillory argues in "Dalilah's House," Milton identifies himself in *Samson Agonistes* with the embattled and marginalized Galileo, in book 8 his specific concern, as I will argue, is with the role that astronomy and natural philosophy would play in England in undergirding the privileges of the monarch and the landed elite.

8. See Jacob, *Henry Stubbe.*

9. Boyle, *The Excellency of Theology*, 118.

10. Boyle, *Certain Physiological Essays*, 78.

11. See Markley, *Fallen Languages*, 34–62.

12. Milton, *Complete Poems*, 738–39.

13. For an overview of Wilkins's involvement in the Royal Society, see Shapiro, *John Wilkins*, 191–223.

14. Ibid., 35.

15. Wilkins, *A Discourse Concerning the Beauty of Providence*, n.p.

16. Ibid., 85, 127.

17. Wilkins, *The Beauty of Providence*, 134–35. Wilkins offers similar counsel in *Of the Principles and Duties of Natural Religion* (London, 1675), in which he pronounces that "general success . . . in the ordinary course of things doth accompany honest and virtuous actions." His confidence in the just order of nature and of life under the restored monarchy is clear in his assertion that "Both *Virtue* and Vice [are] generally and for the most part, sufficiently distinguished by Rewards and Punishments in this life" (85).

18. Shapiro, *John Wilkins*, 70; Wilkins, *The Beauty of Providence*, 83.

19. Shapiro, *John Wilkins*, 29, 70, 150.

20. Wilkins, *Discovery of a World*, 39–40, 52.

21. Wilkins, *Natural Religion*, 409.

22. Ross, *The New Planet No Planet*, 117.

23. All citations from *Paradise Lost* are from Milton, *Complete Poems and Major Prose.*

24. Joseph Wittreich observes in "Inspir'd with Contradiction" that for Milton, truth in the postlapsarian world is always "partial, limited, relative [and] contingent" (158); it is in this context, he observes, that Milton approaches the debates concerning cosmological order.

25. Wilkins, *Discovery of a World*, 120, 190.

26. Ibid., 28–29, 119, 205.

27. Ibid., 207–8.

28. Stillman, *New Philosophy*, 239, 243.

29. Lewalski, "Milton and the Hartlib Circle," 216.

30. I agree with Diane McColley's argument in "Beneficent Hierarchies" that book 8 asserts an environmental ethic of stewardship and explores the hierarchical relationship of Adam and Eve and humans and nature as interrelated concerns. McColley's reading, however, overlooks the range of responses that Eve articulates to the natural world and renders her the unproblematic spokesperson for an environmental ethic of reverence and restraint.

31. Schoenfeldt, "Gender and Conduct in *Paradise Lost*," 319; see also Schoenfeldt, "Among Unequals What Society."

32. In "Milton and the Hartlib Circle" Lewalski elucidates the limits of the egalitarian rhetoric of the Hartlib circle, noting that their projects "often had the stated design of promoting intellectual uniformity" (207). Milton's "deepest conviction," she states, "is that genuine education (and especially higher education) must be largely self-motivated and self-directed. He has no faith in perfect methods or systems nor in epitomes or encyclopedias" (205–6).

33. Achinstein, *Milton and the Revolutionary Reader*.

34. McRae, *God Speed the Plough*, esp. 135–68.

35. DuRocher, "Careful Plowing." McRae's consideration of the range of ideologies associated with the ploughman figure in *Paradise Lost* complicates DuRocher's argument that the figure demonstrates Milton's sympathy with the Diggers. My own reading of Milton's politics is somewhat more conservative.

35. Milton, *Complete Poems*, 634, 635.

36. Wilding, *Dragon's Teeth*, 24. Peter Lindenbaum has recently asserted, in fact, that "Milton's particular achievement or distinction was to construct the most uncontemplative Paradise in the whole hexameral tradition" ("John Milton and the Republican Mode of Literary Production," 159). My reading of Milton's treatment of labor and of his relationship to an emergent capitalist economy differs significantly from that of Nancy Armstrong and Leonard Tennenhouse in *The Imaginary Puritan: Literature, Intellectual Labor, and the Origins of Personal Life* (Berkeley and Los Angeles: U of California P, 1992), 89–113, who view Milton as unproblematically valorizing intellectual over manual labor and overlook the extent to which Milton implicates an emergent capitalism economy in his critique of luxury and an ethos of leisure and consumption.

37. Blith, *The English Improver Improved*, n.p., 2; Hartlib, Samuel Hartlib, *His Legacy of Husbandry*, 139. Blith's ostensible attempts to distance himself from the radical claims and practices of the Diggers may, in fact, be read as signaling his sympathy for their goals:

Although I indeavor so mainly to work my Improvements out of the Belly of the Earth, yet am I neither of the Diggers mind, nor shall I imitate their practice, for though the poor are or ought to have advantage upon the Commons, yet I question whether they as a society gathered together from all parts of the Nation could claim a right to any particular Common: And for their prastice [*sic*], if there be not thousands of places more capable of Improvement than theirs, and that by many easier waies, and to far greater advantages, I will lay down the Bucklers: Nor shal I countenance the Level principles of Parity or Equality, which they seem to urge from the beginning till I see the heads of Families and Tribes, Judges and Governors, Lords and Princes of whole Countries, blotted out from the first or succeeding generation; unless they bring us to the new *Jerusalem*, or bring it down to us, when we shall not need to trouble our selves about greater or lesser, or any distinction of person, places, or estates, any more, but this Parity is all I endeavor, to make the poor rich, and the rich richer, and all to live of the labour of their own hands.

If, for the present, Blith seems content to "make the poor rich, and the rich richer," he seems nonetheless sympathetic to the goals of the Diggers' millenarian project. His disagreements with the Diggers seem to stem more from the logistical problems he identifies with their project than from any sense of ideological revulsion at the prospect of erasing the "troubl[ing] distinctions of person, places, or estates" (n.p.).

38. Sharrock, *History*, n.p.; Evelyn, *Sylva*, n.p. Another example of the elitism of the Royal Society's studies in husbandry is found in John Beale's *Herefordshire Orchards: A Pattern for All England* (1657), in which the "common husbandmen" who "keep their small flocks at all adventure without much care or caution" come under repeated attack.

39. Boyle, *Some Considerations*, n.p.

40. Ibid., 30.

41. Boyle, *Excellency of Theology*, n.p.

42. Rogers nevertheless sees evidence of Milton's retreat from the most radical implications of his onistic vitalism in the imagery of the purging of the "tartareous dregs" in book 8, ll. 233–41 (*The Matter of Revolution*, esp. 132–43).

43. On women's exclusion from the institutions of science in the seventeenth century and the implications for the interpretation of nature and the body, see Schiebinger, *The Mind Has No Sex?*, and Merchant, *The Death of Nature*. On women's quest for participation in the discourses of natural philosophy, astronomy, and medicine in the seventeenth and eighteenth centuries, see Parker, *The Scientific Lady*, 5–180. On Milton and gender, see Wilding, "Thir Sex Not Equal Seem'd"; Radzinowicz, "Milton on the Tragic Women of Genesis"; Wittreich, "Inspir'd with Contradiction"; Lieb, "Two of Far Nobler Shape"; Parisi, "Discourse and Danger."

44. Margaret Cavendish is one of the few women known to have succeeded in securing a single, and evidently brief, visit to the laboratory of the Royal Society; her nickname "Mad Madge" is an indication of the ridicule that was heaped upon women like Cavendish who challenged the exclusively male preserves of learning and debate.

45. McColley, however, overlooks in "Beneficent Hierarchies" the coercive implications of Eve's subsequent arguments for an aggressive program for "improving" the Garden.

46. See Guillory, "From the Superfluous to the Supernumerary," and McColley, "Beneficent Hierarchy." My reading of Milton's treatment of the gendered hierarchy of book 8 is substantially closer to McColley's than to Guillory's. McColley sees "Paradisal hierarchies" as "beneficent, flexible, and reciprocal" (232). Guillory's reading fails to acknowledge both the complex relationship between astronomy and theology in the period, and the extent to which seventeenth-century astronomy is shaped by, and continues to authorize, gendered assumptions. He sees Milton's apparent dismissal of astronomy as motivated by the ostensible recognition that in the seventeenth century, gender is already a "charming poeticism of a prescientific discourse"; as such, he represents the poet as retreating into theology in order to authorize the subordinate status of woman. He overlooks the ways in which Raphael challenges and tempers Adam's coercive construction of gender in book 8. Guillory also underestimates the extent to which gendered assumptions continue to permeate and shape a broad range of scientific discourses and practices; he sees these assumptions as largely confined to "medical practices, hygienic programs, and psychological therapies" (83).

47. Wilkins, *Discourse*, 80, 203–204, cited in McColley; *Discovery*, 75–76, 77.

48. See Radzinowicz, "Politics of *Paradise Lost*"; Wilding, "Thir Sex Not Equal Seem'd"; Wilding, *Dragon's Teeth*, esp. 205–58; and Stephen M. Buhler, "Kingly

States: The Politics in *Paradise Lost*," *Milton Studies* 32 (1995): 49–68; all three authors argue that meritocracy is, for Milton, the divinely sanctioned model of human governance. As Buhler has observed, God's insistence that Christ is "Found worthiest to be so by being Good,/Far more than Great or High" (3:310–11) sanctions meritocracy as the ideal form of government, while Satan articulates a model of tyranny in his suggestion that the angels were "ordain'd to govern, not to serve" (5:802). In book 7, Adam's condemnation of Nimrod and the political logic leading to the construction of the tower of Babel is yet more pointed. "Man over men/[God] made not Lord; such title to himself/ Reserving, human left from human free" (69–71). As Wilding observes, the emphasis Milton places on individual rights and liberty demonstrates the persistence of his radical commitments well into the Restoration (*Dragon's Teeth*, 248).

49. Wilding, "Thir Sex Not Equal Seem'd," 185.

50. Rajan's reading in "Banyan Trees and Fig Leaves" concurs in some essential points with David Quint's in *Epic and Empire*. For a more ambivalent reading of colonialism and Paradise Lost, see Stevens, "*Paradise Lost* and the Colonial Imperative."

51. Merchant, *The Death of Nature*, 39. Albanese suggests that despite Milton's ostensible demonization of novelty, optical devices nevertheless anachronistically intrude themselves into the text. "The occasional play of optical devices in the text presents the alternative, the artificial body of the scientific project as an inadvertent critique" of the mortal, postlapsarian body (*New Science*, 125). This passage is, however, only one of many in *Paradise Lost* in which the poet implicitly scrutinizes and critiques the coercive uses of prosthetic technologies, which for both Milton and Donne simply "perfect" the strategies of domination and subjugation that define the exercise of power in the postlapsarian world. For a reading that concurs with my own and treats this issue in depth, see Boesky, "Milton, Galileo, and Sunspots."

52. Milton, *Complete Poems*, 296, 606.

53. U.S. Senate Committee on Labor and Human Resources, *Oversight of the Healthy Start Demonstration Project*, 4–5.

Chapter 4. "The Threatning Angel and the Speaking Ass"

1. Schiebinger, *The Mind Has No Sex?*, 15.

2. In 1701 the poem appeared in Charles Gildon's *Miscellany* (London). In 1709 it was reprinted along with "A Prospect of Death" in a slim volume attributed

to that ubiquitous anonymous "Lady." Finch citations are drawn here from
Reynolds, *The Poems of Anne, Countess of Winchilsea*, which includes a version of
"The Spleen" published in the 1713 edition of Finch's *Miscellany Poems* and, as
such, reflects the poet's own final revisions of the work. My own decision to
preserve the original irregular spelling is in part a response to the remarks of
John Middleton Murry in his edition *Poems by Anne Finch, Countess of Winchilsea,
1661–1720* (London: Jonathan Cape, 1928). Murray, who regularized the spelling
of the poem, states that the "old and obsolete spelling and punctuation" of the
1713 edition "interpose a veil between him [the reader] and the object, so that the
impression made upon him by the poetry is never direct and definite. Therefore,
he grows weary of the attempt to force a contact with it" (3). The remarks
convinced me that Finch's idiosyncratic spelling and punctuation are perfectly in
keeping with my own reading of the poem.

3. McGovern, *Anne Finch*, esp. 159–78, and Hinnant, *The Poetry of Anne Finch,*
esp. 197–226. Both recognize, to varying degrees, the ideological operation of the
discourses of the spleen. An earlier study by Katherine Rogers, "Finch's 'Candid
Account' vs. Eighteenth-Century Theories of the Spleen," *Mosaic* 22 (1989):
17–27, focuses on the "scientific" accuracy of Finch's account of the spleen.

4. McGovern, *Anne Finch*, 160.

5. Hinnant, *The Poetry of Anne Finch*, 198.

6. On the experimental interests of physicians in the seventeenth century, see
Frank, "The Physician as Virtuoso"; on Harvey's impact on seventeenth-century
physiology and experimental method, see also Frank, *Harvey and the Oxford Physi-
ologists*, and Webster, *The Great Instauration*, esp. 315–23.

7. Trotter, *The Poetry of Abraham Cowley*, 116.

8. Sprat, *History of the Royal Society*, 44.

9. Cowley, *Poetry and Prose*, xi.

10. See McGovern's discussion of "The Introduction" in *Anne Finch*, 124–27.

11. Addison referred to the spleen as "*le spleen anglais*," calling it "a kind of
demon that haunts the nation" (cited in Porter, *Mind-Forg'd Manacles*, 81). George
Cheyne dubbed the phenomenon the "English Malady." In his writings on hysteria
and hypochondria, Sydenham classified the phenomena as epidemic diseases.

12. See Mullan, "Hypochondria and Hysteria," and Mullan, *Sentiment and Sensibility,*
201–40. On the class-specific nature of the spleen, see also Porter, *Mind Forg'd
Manacles*, 81–87. "The inactivity and sedentary Occupations of the better Sort
(among whom this evil most rages)" numbered, for George Cheyne, among the

several causes of the spleen (*The English Malady*, I; see also the section entitled "The English Malady as a Disease of Civilization" (xxvi–xxxii in Porter's extensive introduction). Porter observes that for Cheyne, as for other specialists in the spleen, "Nervous disorders constituted authentic physical diseases, causing profound suffering," yet they were the price of progress as much as the wages of sin. Attacking the prosperous, they were the marks of distinction, a success tax on a busy hive buzzing as never before—urban, affluent, aspiring and ambitious" (*Mind Forg'd Manacles*, 83).

13. Sydenham, *The Whole Works*, 455.

14. In *Of the Spleen* (1723) William Stukeley wrote that "the modish disease call'd the vapors . . . from its suppos'd seat, the SPLEEN, does most frequently attack scholars and persons of the soft sex most eminent for wit and good sense" (25). Addressing Cheyne in a letter in 1734, David Hume suggests that the "inflam'd Imaginations" engendered by the Spleen spurred the course of his "Philosophical Enquiries" and associates his medical predicament with a long tradition of philosophers who have been "overthrown by the Greatness of their Genius" (*Letters*, 16). He strongly suggests, moreover, that Cheyne's confirms the good doctor's own genius, since it had gone undetected by others "unacquainted with these Motions of the Mind" (18). He concludes his letter by inquiring as to how long he will have to "endure the Fatigue of deep & abstruse thinking" (18).

15. Markley, "Sentimentality as Performance," 212.

16. Willis, *The London Practice of Physick*, 297–98.

17. Sydenham, *The Whole Works*, 441.

18. Cunningham, "Thomas Sydenham," 180, 189. Sydenham's early association with Boyle lent fuel to the attacks on the Royal Society by Henry Stubbe, who observed that with the exception of Sydenham and Boyle's physician Thomas Coxe, "not one [physician] lives that doth not condemn your experimental philosophy" (cited in ibid., 180–81).

19. Dewhurst makes this claim in *Dr. Thomas Sydenham*, 62, but unfortunately does not cite his source.

20. Cited in Cunningham, "Thomas Sydenham," 181.

21. Cunningham, "Thomas Sydenham," 170, 177.

22. Sydenham, *The Whole Works*, 446. In a letter to his longtime patient Samuel Richardson, Cheyne writes: "You are a true genuine Hyppo now with all its plainest Symptoms. . . . the Course, the Obstinacy of this Distemper is as various

as the Faces, Complexions and original Frame of each individual are. It is called a true Proteus and is never to be reduced into particular Rules" (*The Letters of Dr. George Cheyne to Samuel Richardson [1733–1743]*, ed. Charles F. Mullett [New York: Columbia University Press, 1943], 104, cited in Stephenson, "Richardson's 'Nerves'"). Richardson's condition is tailor-made for him by Cheyne: the symptoms are as unique as his own personality—in fact, indistinguishable from it. Cheyne, in effect, diagnoses Richardson as an anomolous free agent in an increasingly mechanical universe.

23. Markley, "Sentimentality as Performance," 212.

24. Sydenham, *The Whole Works*, 440, 465, 447.

25. In his *Treatise of the Hypochondriack and Hysterick Passions* (London, 1711), Bernard de Mandeville's literary persona suggests that women are inherently more frail than men both intellectually and physically, and therefore more prone to hysteria:

We are of a stronger, but they of a more Elegant composure, and Beauty is their attribute as Strength is ours: Their frame, tho less firm is more delicate, and themselves more capable of Pleasure and of Pain, tho' endued with less constancy of bearing the excess of either. This delicacy, as well as imbecillity of the Spirits in Women is Conspicuous in all their actions, those of the Brain not excepted. They are unfit both for abstruse and elaborate Thoughts, all Studies of Depth, Coherence, and Solidity that fatigue the Spirits, and require a steadiness and assiduity of thinking, but where the Advantages of Education and Knowledge are equal, [women] exceed the Men in Sprightliness of Fancy, quickness of Thought and offhand Wit; as much as they out-do them in sweetness of Voice and Volubility of Tongue" (175).

De Mandeville's deterministic physiology of femininity becomes an argument to counter the vocal calls of feminist polemicists for educational equality. Equal education, de Mandeville suggests, cannot compensate for the natural "delicacy" of women's intellectual faculties, or render women capable of "Studies of Depth," or serious intellectual pursuits. It will, in fact, only serve the same function that the limited education of bourgeois women presently serves, which is to equip her to provide diverting conversation for her spouse, a skill that will complement her other essential natural attribute: beauty. The passage reflects, moreover, the suspicion of feminine sexuality that is inseparable from the idea of hysteria. As Mullan has suggested, it is precisely the "tenderness" and sensitivity of women that "disposes them 'to be Hysterick'" (*Sentiment and Sensibility*, 218). The acute sensitivity of women's bodies, de Mandeville suggests, renders them susceptible to excesses of passion—specifically, to sexual excess.

26. Sydenham, *The Whole Works*, 451. Cheyne explicitly associates the spleen with effeminacy. The Greeks, he suggests, should serve as a warning to the British: "in Proportion as they advanced in Learning, and the Knowledge of the Sciences, and distinguished themselves from other Nations by their Politeness and Refinement, they sunk into *Effeminacy, Luxury,* and *Diseases*" (*English Malady,* xxviii). Sydenham does caution against the dangers of overbleeding female patients: while himself prescribing that as much as eight ounces of blood be let at a time, his example of the dangers of overbleeding involves a "vertuous Matron of good Quality" who dies because of the "mischief [and] over-Officiousness" of the women attending her, who, in Sydenham's absence and against his orders, had "a vein opened" in her ankle (474).

27. I am drawing here on McGovern's argument that the poem associates the discourse of the spleen with a "Puritan obsession with sin and the emphasis on repression" that is ostensibly "inimical to her Anglican faith" (*Anne Finch,* 177).

28. Mullan, *Sentiment and Sensibility,* 224; Sydenham, *The Whole Works,* 467.

29. Ibid., 445.

30. My reading of these lines differs significantly from McGovern's, who sees the lines as providing evidence of Finch's illness. She argues that "Her horror at the effects of the spleen is due to her awareness that such distorted judgment of her own verse and about what others think of it is a paranoia resulting from the illness and runs counter to reality" (*Anne Finch,* 172).

31. Citations of poems by Tollet and Montagu are from Lonsdale, ed., *The New Oxford Book of Eighteenth-Century Verse.*

32. Sydenham, *The Whole Works,* 439. Finch's maneuver undermines the oppositional relationship Cowley enshrines in "To the Royal Society" between the feminine "Diserts of Poetry" and the "solid Meats" of empirical data that are needed to "increase [the] force" of an authoritative and conspicuously masculine natural philosophy. Poetry, Cowley suggests, leads only into the "pleasant Labyrinths of ever-fresh Discourse," through "painted Scenes, and Pageants of the Brain," while natural philosophy will yield definitive truths, "carrying [man] to see/The Riches which do hoorded for him lye" in the "endless Treasury" of feminized nature. Cowley's rhetoric discloses the imperialist ambitions that fueled and shaped the interests and activities of the experimentalists. The "great Champions" of natural philosophy, he suggests, will provide the means of exploiting the natural resources of those "spacious Countrys."

33. Robert Frank observes that Lower was apparently distinguished by his fondness for dissection and vivisection; on the use of vivisection by Lower and

other members of the Royal Society, see *Harvey and the Oxford Physiologists*, esp. 171–205. See also Guerrini, "The Ethics of Animal Experimentation." One particularly famous experiment in which Lower participated, also documented by Frank, involved "keeping a dog alive by the mechanical means of a bellows while cutting away the dog's thorax and diaphragm to observe the exposed beating heart" (400). After participating in the experiment for the first time, Hooke observed in a letter to Boyle, "I shall hardly be induced to make any further trials of this kind, because of the torture of the creature: but certainly the enquiry would be very noble, if we could find any way to stupify the creature, as it might not be sensible, which I fear there is hardly an opiate will perform." Guerrini notes that "At about the same time, in his *Micrographia*, Hooke commented that the microscope beneficially empowered one to look at nature 'acting according to her usual course and way, undisturbed, whereas, when we endeavor to pry into her secrets by opening the doors upon her, and dissecting and mangling creatures whil'st there is life yet within them, we find her indeed at work, but put into such disorder by the violence offer'd that the accuracy of our observations is put in doubt'" (401). Similarly, Finch suggests that the male physician elicits the symptoms of disorder he describes in his female patients.

34. Rogers and McCarthy, *Meridian Anthology*, 102.

35. McGovern, *Anne Finch*, 174.

36. See Catherine Gallagher, "Embracing the Absolute: The Politics of the Female Subject in Seventeenth-Century England," *Genders* 1 (1988): 24–39.

37. See Salvaggio, *Enlightened Absence*, 11–18. On the gender politics of psychoanalysis and hysteria, see also Bernheimer, ed., *In Dora's Case*, and Catherine Clement, "The Guilty One."

39. The lines may also allude to Cowley's implicit dismissal of Philips's talent as anomalous among women: "Of all the Female race," writes Cowley in "On the Death of Mrs. Katherine Philips," "This is the Sovereign Face."

40. Sydenham, *The Whole Works*, 455.

Afterword

1. Haraway, *Simians, Cyborgs, and Women*, 199.

2. See Hill, *The World Turned Upside Down*; Hill, *The Century of Revolution, 1603–1714* (New York: Norton, 1980); Hill, *Change and Continuity in Seventeenth-Century England* (New Haven, Conn.: Yale UP, 1991); Nigel Smith, ed., *A Collection*

of Ranter Writings from the Seventeenth-Century; Smith, *Literature and Revolution in England, 1640–1660;* Mack, *Visionary Women.*

3. Bacon, *Works* 3:294.

4. See Proctor, esp. "'Doubt Is Our Product': Trade Association Science," in *Cancer Wars,* 101–32.

WORKS CITED

Achinstein, Sharon. *Milton and the Revolutionary Reader*. Princeton, N.J.: Princeton UP, 1994.

Adams, Hazard. "One Direction for Donne's Skepticism." M.A. thesis. University of Washington, 1949.

Aers, David, and Gunther Kress. "'Dark Texts Need Notes': Versions of Self in Donne's Verse Epistles." In *Critical Essays on John Donne*, ed. Arthur Marotti, 102–22. New York: G. K. Hall, 1994.

Albanese, Denise. *New Science, New World*. Durham, N.C., Duke UP, 1996.

Armstrong, Nancy, and Leonard Tennenhouse. *The Imaginary Puritan: Literature, Intellectual Labor, and the Origins of Personal Life*. Berkeley and Los Angeles: U of California P, 1992.

Augustine. *On Christian Doctrine*. Ed. D. W. Robertson Jr. Indianapolis: Bobbs-Merrill, 1958.

Bacon, Francis. *The Essayes of Francis Bacon*. Ed. Richard Whately. New York, 1857.

———. *The Letters and the Life of Francis Bacon*. Ed. James Spedding. 7 vols. London, 1861–74.

———. *The Wisedome of the Ancients* (1609). Trans. Sir Arthur Gorges. London, 1619. Facsimile reprint. New York: Garland, 1976.

———. *The Works of Francis Bacon*. Ed. J. Spedding, R. L. Ellis, D. D. Heath. 7 vols. London, 1857–61.

Bald, R. C. *John Donne: A Life*. Oxford: Oxford UP, 1970.

———. *Donne and the Drurys*. Cambridge: Cambridge UP, 1959.

Batt, Sharon. *Patient No More: The Politics of Breast Cancer*. Charlottetown, Prince Edward Island, Canada: Synergy Books, 1994.

Baumgaertner, Jill Peláez. "Political Play and Theological Uncertainty in the Anniversaries." *John Donne Journal* 13 (1994): 29–49.

Beale, John. *Herefordshire Orchards: A Pattern for All England.* London, 1657.

Belsey, Catherine. *John Milton, Language, Gender, Power.* Oxford: Basil Blackwell, 1988.

Benet, Diana Trevino. "Sexual Transgression in Donne's Elegies." *Modern Philology* 92 (1994): 14–35.

Bernheimer, Charles, ed. *In Dora's Case: Freud—Hysteria—Feminism.* New York: Columbia UP, 1985.

Bewley, Marius. "Religious Cynicism in Donne's Poetry." *Kenyon Review* 14 (1952): 619–46.

Biagioli, Mario. *Galileo, Courtier: The Practice of Science in the Culture of Absolutism.* Chicago: U of Chicago P, 1993.

————. "Galileo's System of Patronage." *History of Science* 28 (1990): 1–62.

————. "Galileo the Emblem-Maker." *Isis* 28 (1990): 1–62.

Blith, Walter. *The English Improver Improved, or The Survey of Husbandry Surveyed.* 1649. 3rd ed. London, 1653.

Boesky, Amy. "Milton, Galileo, and Sunspots: Optics and Uncertainty in *Paradise Lost.*" *Milton Studies* 34 (1996): 23–43.

Bono, James J. *The Word of God and the Languages of Man: Interpreting Nature in Early Modern Science and Medicine.* Madison: U of Wisconsin P, 1995.

Boyle, Robert. *Certain Physiological Essays.* London, 1661.

————. *The Excellence of Theology, as Compar'd with Natural Philosophy.* London, 1674.

————. *Some Considerations Touching the Usefulness of Experimental Natural Philosophy.* 1663. 2nd ed. Oxford, 1664.

Breitenberg, Mark. *Anxious Masculinity in Early Modern England.* New York: Cambridge UP, 1996.

Briggs, John C. *Francis Bacon and the Rhetoric of Nature.* Cambridge, Mass.: Harvard UP, 1989.

Bryant, Bunyan, and Paul Mohai, eds. *Race and the Incidence of Environmental Hazards: A Time for Discourse.* Boulder, Colo.: Westview Press, 1992.

Buhler, Stephen M. "Kingly States: The Politics in *Paradise Lost.*" *Milton Studies* 32 (1995): 49–68.

Bullard, Robert. *Dumping in Dixie: Race, Class and Environmental Quality.* Boulder, Colo.: Westview Press, 1990.

————, ed. *Unequal Protection, Environmental Justice, and Communities of Color.* San Francisco: Sierra Club Books, 1994.

Burtt, E. A. *The Metaphysical Foundations of Modern Science.* 2d ed. London: Routledge & Kegan Paul, 1934.

Carey, John. *John Donne: Life, Mind and Art.* London: Oxford UP, 1980.

Carson, Rachel. *Silent Spring.* 1962. Reprint. Boston: Houghton Mifflin, 1994.

Cheyne, George. *The English Malady* (1733). Ed. Roy Porter. London: Tavistock Routledge, 1991.

Cixous, Hélène. "Sorties." In *The Newly Born Woman,* trans. Betsy Wing. Theory and History of Literature, vol. 24. Minneapolis: U of Minnesota P, 1986.

Clement, Catherine. "The Guilty One." In *The Newly Born Woman,* trans. Betsy Wing. Minneapolis: U of Minnesota P, 1986.

Cobbett, William. *A Complete Collection of State Trials.* 21 vols. London, 1809–14.

Coffin, Charles Monroe. *John Donne and the New Philosophy.* 1937. Reprint. New York: Humanities Press, 1958.

Colborn, Theodora, Dianne Dumonoski, and John Peterson Myers. *Our Stolen Future: Are We Threatening Our Fertility, Intelligence and Survival?* New York: Dutton, 1996.

Cormack, Leslie B. "Twisting the Lion's Tail: Practice and Theory in the Court of Henry Prince of Wales." In *Patronage and Institutions: Science, Technology, and Medicine at the European Court, 1500–1700,* ed. Bruce T. Moran, 67–84. Rochester, N.Y.: Boydell Press, 1991.

Cowley, Abraham. *Poetry and Prose, with Thomas Sprat's Life and Observations by Dryden, Addison, Johnson and Others.* Ed. L. C. Martin. Oxford: Oxford UP, 1949.

———. *The Works of Abraham Cowley.* London, 1668.

Cunningham, Andrew. "Thomas Sydenham: Epidemics, Experiment and the 'Good Old Cause.'" In *The Medical Revolution of the Seventeenth-Century,* ed. Roger French and Andrew Wear, 164–90. Cambridge: Cambridge UP, 1989.

Dewhurst, Kenneth. *Dr. Thomas Sydenham, 1624–1689: His Life and Writings.* Berkeley and Los Angeles: U of California P, 1966.

Docherty, Thomas. *John Donne Undone.* New York: Methuen, 1986.

Dollimore, Jonathan, *Radical Tragedy: Religion, Ideology, and Power in the Drama of Shakespeare and His Contemporaries.* Chicago: U of Chicago P, 1984.

Donne, John. *Biathanatos.* Ed. John William Hebel. New York: Facsimile Text Society, 1930.

———. *The Complete English Poems.* Ed. C. A. Patrides. 1985. Reprint. London: Everyman, 1994.

———. *The Complete Poetry and Selected Prose of John Donne.* Ed. Charles Monroe Coffin. 1941. Reprint. New York: Modern Library, 1994.

————. *The Courtier's Library, or Catalogus Librorum Aulicorum.* Ed. Evelyn M. Simpson. Soho: Nonesuch Press, 1930.

————. *Essays in Divinity.* Ed. Evelyn M. Simpson. Oxford: Oxford UP, 1952.

————. *Ignatius His Conclave.* Ed. Timothy Healy. Oxford: Oxford UP, 1969.

————. *Pseudo-Martyr: Wherein Out of Certain Propositions and Gradations, This Conclusion Is Euicted: That Those Which Are of the Romane Religion in This Kingdome, May and Ought to Take the Oath of Allegiance.* London, 1610.

————. *Sermons of John Donne.* Ed. R. Potter and Evelyn Simpson. 10 vols. Berkeley and Los Angeles: U of California P, 1953–62.

————. *The Variorum Edition of the Poetry of John Donne.* Ed. Gary A. Stringer. 6 vols. Bloomington: Indiana UP, 1995.

Dubrow, Heather. *Echoes of Desire: English Petrarchism and Its Counterdiscourses.* Ithaca, N.Y.: Cornell UP, 1995.

————. "'The Sun in Water': Donne's Somerset Epithalamium and the Poetics of Patronage." In *The Historical Renaissance: New Essays on Tudor and Stuart Literature and Culture,* ed. Heather Dubrow and Richard Strier, 197–219. Chicago: U of Chicago P, 1988.

DuRocher, Richard J. "Careful Plowing: Culture and Agriculture in *Paradise Lost.*" *Milton Studies* 31 (1994): 91–107.

Easlea, Brian. *Witch Hunting, Magic and the New Philosophy: An Introduction to Debates of the Scientific Revolution, 1450–1750.* Sussex: Harvester press, 1980.

Elliot, Ralph W. V. "Isaac Newton's 'Of an Universall Language." *Modern Language Review* 52 (1957): 1–18.

Elsky, Martin. *Authorizing Words: Speech, Writing, and Print in the English Renaissance.* Ithaca, N.Y.: Cornell UP, 1989.

————. "Bacon's Hieroglyphics and the Separation of Words and Things." *Philological Quarterly* 63 (1984): 449–60.

Estrin, Barbara. *Laura: Uncovering Gender and Genre in Wyatt, Donne, and Marvell.* Durham, N.C.: Duke UP, 1994.

Evelyn, John. *Sylva, or A Discourse of Forest-Trees and the Propagation of Timber in His Majesties Dominions.* 1664. 2nd ed. London, 1670.

Finch, Anne. *The Poems of Anne, Countess of Winchilsea.* Ed. Myra Reynolds. Chicago: U of Chicago P, 1909.

————. *Poems by Anne Finch, Countess of Winchilsea, 1661–1720.* Ed. John Middleton Murry. London: Jonathan Cape, 1928.

Fish, Stanley. *Surprized by Sin: The Reader in Paradise Lost.* New York: St. Martin's Press, 1967.

Foucault, Michel. *Discipline and Punish: The Birth of the Prison.* Trans. Alan Sheridan. New York: Pantheon Books, 1977.

———. *Madness and Civilization: A History of Madness in the Age of Reason.* Trans. Richard Howard. New York: Pantheon Books, 1965.

Frank, Robert F., Jr. *Harvey and the Oxford Physiologist: A Study of Scientific Ideas.* Berkeley and Los Angeles: U of California P, 1980.

———. "The Physician as Virtuoso in Seventeenth-Century England." In *English Scientific Virtuosi in the Sixteenth and Seventeenth Centuries,* ed. Barbara Shapiro and Robert Frank Jr., 59–103. Los Angeles: Clark Library, 1979.

Galilei, Galileo. *Siderius nuncius, or The Sidereal Messenger.* Trans. Albert an Helden. Chicago: Chicago UP, 1989.

Gilbert, Sandra, and Susan Gubar. *The Madwoman in the Attic: The Woman Writer and the Nineteenth-Century Literary Imagination.* New Haven, Conn.: Yale UP, 1979.

Gilden, Charles. *Miscellany Poems.* London, 1701.

Gleason, J. B. "Dr. Donne in the Court of Kings: A Glimpse from Marginalia." *Journal of English and Germanic Philology* 69 (1970): 599–612.

Gottlieb, Robert. *Forcing the Spring: The Transformation of the American Environmental Movement.* Washington, D.C.: Island Press, 1993.

Gould, Stephen J. *The Mismeasure of Man.* New York: Norton, 1981.

Greenblatt, Stephen. *Renaissance Self-Fashioning from More to Shakespeare.* Chicago: U of Chicago P, 1980.

Guerrini, Anita. "The Ethics of Animal Experimentation in Seventeenth-Century England." *Journal of the History of Ideas* 50 (1989): 391–407.

Guibbory, Achsah. "Donne, Milton, and Holy Sex." *Milton Studies* 32 (1995): 3–21.

———. "'Oh, Let Mee Not Serve So': The Politics of Love in Donne's *Elegies.*" In *Critical Essays on John Donne,* ed. Arthur Marotti, 17–36. New York: Macmillan, 1994.

Guillory, John. "Dalilah's House: *Samson Agonistes* and the Sexual Division of Labor." In *Rewriting the Renaissance: The Discourse of Sexual Difference in Early Modern Europe,* ed. Margaret W. Ferguson, Maureen Quilligan, and Nancy J. Vickers, 106–22. Chicago: U of Chicago P, 1986.

———. "From the Superfluous to the Supernumerary: Reading Gender in *Paradise Lost.*" In *Soliciting Interpretation: Literary Theory and Seventeenth-Century English Poetry,* ed. Elizabeth D. Harvey and Katherine Eisaman Maus, 68–88. Chicago: U of Chicago P, 1990.

Hacking, Ian. *The Emergence of Probability: A Philosophical Study of Early Ideas about Probability, Induction and Statistical Inference.* Cambridge: Cambridge UP, 1975.

Hall, Joseph. *The Works of the Right Reverend Father in God Joseph Hall, Lord Bishop of Norwich.* 1647. London, 1714.

Haraway, Donna. *Simians, Cyborgs, and Women: The Reinvention of Nature.* New York: Routledge, 1991.

Harland, Paul. "Donne's Political Intervention in the Parliament of 1629." *John Donne Journal* 11 (1992): 21–38.

Harris, Victor. *All Coherence Gone.* Chicago: U of Chicago P, 1949.

Hartlib, Samuel. *Samuel Hartlib, His Legacy of Husbandry.* 1647. 3rd ed. London, 1655.

Hawarde, John. *Les Reportes del Cases in Camera Stellata, 1593–1609.* Ed. W. P. Baildon. London, 1894.

Haydn, Hiram. *The Counter-Renaissance.* New York: Scribner, 1950.

Helgerson, Richard. *Forms of Nationhood: The Elizabethan Writing of England.* Chicago: U of Chicago P, 1992.

Hill, Christopher. *The Collected Essays of Christopher Hill.* Vol. 2. Amherst: U of Massachusetts P, 1986.

———. *Milton and the English Revolution.* 1977. Reprint. New York: Penguin Books, 1979.

———. *The World Turned Upside Down: Radical Ideas during the English Revolution.* 1972. Reprint. New York: Penguin Books, 1982.

Hinnant, Charles. *The Poetry of Anne Finch: An Essay in Interpretation.* Newark: U of Delaware P, 1994.

Historical Manuscripts Commission, London. *Reports and Papers.* Hastings MSS, IV.

Hofrichter, Richard, ed. *Toxic Struggles: The Theory and Practice of Environmental Justice.* Philadelphia: New Society, 1993.

Hume, David. *The Letters of David Hume.* Ed. J. Y. T. Grieg. Oxford: Clarendon Press, 1932.

Hunt, William. "The Spectral Origins of the English Revolution." In *Reviving the English Revolution,* ed. Geoff Eley and William Hunt, 304–32. London: Verso, 1988.

Hurley, Andrew. *Environmental Inequalities: Class, Race, and Industrial Pollution in Gary, Indiana, 1945–80.* Chapel Hill: U of North Carolina P, 1995.

Irigaray, Luce. "Is the Subject of Science Sexed?" *Cultural Critique* 1 (1985): 73–88.

Jacob, J. R. *Henry Stubbe, Radical Protestantism and the Early Enlightenment.* Cambridge: Cambridge UP, 1983.

———. "Restoration Ideologies and the Royal Society." *History of Science* 17 (1980): 25–38.

———. "Restoration, Reformation and the Origins of the Royal Society." *History of Science* 13 (1975): 155–76.

———. *Robert Boyle and the English Revolution.* New York: Burt Franklin, 1977.

Jacob, J. R., and Margaret C. Jacob. "The Anglican Origins of Modern Science: The Metaphysical Foundations of the Whig Constitution." *Isis* 71 (1980): 117–30.

Jacobus, Lee. *Sudden Apprehension: Aspects of Knowledge in "Paradise Lost."* Paris: Mouton, 1976,.

Jardine, Lisa. *Francis Bacon: Discovery and the Art of Discourse.* Cambridge: Cambridge UP, 1974.

Judson, Margaret. *Crisis of the Constitution: An Essay in Constitutional and Political Thought in England, 1603–1645.* Rutgers, N.J.: Rutgers UP, 1949.

Keller, Evelyn Fox. *Reflections on Gender and Science.* New Haven, Conn.: Yale UP, 1985.

Kerrigan, William. "What Was Donne Doing?" *South Central Review* 4 (1987): 2–15.

Knafla, L. A. *Law and Politics in Jacobean England: The Tracts of Lord Chancellor Ellesmere.* Cambridge: Cambridge UP, 1977.

Knoespel, Kenneth J. "The Emplotment of Chaos: Instability and Narrative Order." In *Chaos and Order: Complex Dynamics in Literature and Science,* ed. N. Katherine Hayles, 100–124. Chicago: U of Chicago P, 1991.

Koyre, Alexander. *From the Closed World to the Infinite Universe.* Baltimore: Johns Hopkins UP, 1957.

Kroll, Richard. *The Material Word: Literate Culture in the Restoration and Early Eighteenth Century.* Baltimore: John Hopkins UP, 1991.

Landry, Donna, and Gerald McLean. "Of Forceps, Patents, and Paternity." *Eighteenth-Century Studies* 23 (1990): 523–43.

Latour, Bruno, and Steve Woolgar. *Laboratory Life: The Social Construction of Scientific Facts.* Princeton, N.J.: Princeton UP, 1986.

Lacqueur, Thomas. *Making Sex: Body and Gender from the Greeks to Freud.* Cambridge, Mass.: Harvard UP, 1990.

Levack, Brian. "Law and Ideology: The Civil Law and Theories of Absolutism in Elizabethan and Jacobean England." In *The Historical Renaissance: New Essays on Tudor and Stuart Literature and Culture,* ed. Heather Dubrow and Richard Strier, 220–41. Chicago: U of Chicago P, 1988.

Lewalski, Barbara. *Donne's "Anniversaries" and the Poetry of Praise: The Creation of the Symbolic Mode.* Princeton, N.J.: Princeton UP, 1973.

———. "Milton and the Hartlib Circle: Educational Projects and Epic Paideia." In *Literary Milton: Text, Pretext, Context,* ed. Diana Trevino Benet and Michael Lieb, 202–19. Pittsburgh: Duquesne UP, 1994.

———. "Milton on Women—Yet Again." In *Problems for Feminist Criticism,* ed. Sally Minogue. New York: Routledge, 1990.

Lieb, Michael. "'Two of Far Nobler Shape': Reading the Paradisal Text." In *Literary Milton: Text, Pretext, Context,* ed. Diana Trevino Benet and Michael Lieb, 114–33. Pittsburgh: Duquesne UP, 1994.

Lindenbaum, Peter. "John Milton and the Republican Mode of Literary Production." In *Critical Essays on John Milton,* ed. Christopher Kendrick, 150–63. New York: G. K. Hall, 1995.

Lonsdale, Roger, ed. *The New Oxford Book of Eighteenth-Century Verse.* Oxford: Oxford UP, 1989.

Lovejoy, Arthur O. "Milton's Dialogue on Astronomy." In *Reason and the Imagination: Studies in the History of Ideas, 1600–1800,* ed. J. A. Mazzeo. New York: Columbia UP, 1962.

McColley, Diane. "Beneficent Hierarchies: Reading Milton Greenly." In *Spokesperson Milton: Voices in Contemporary Criticism,* ed. Charles W. Durham and Kristin Pruitt McColgan, 229–48. Selinsgrove, Pa.: Susquehanna UP, 1994.

McColley, Grant. "Milton's Dialogue on Astronomy: The Principal Immediate Sources." *PMLA* 52 (1937): 728–59.

McGovern, Barbara. *Anne Finch and Her Poetry: A Critical Biography.* Athens: U of George P, 1992.

McRae, Andrew. *God Speed the Plough: The Representation of Agrarian England, 1500–1600.* New York: Cambridge UP, 1996.

Mack, Phyllis. *Visionary Women: Ecstatic Prophesy in Seventeenth-Century England.* Berkeley and Los Angeles: U of California P, 1992.

Mandeville, Bernard de. *Treatise of the Hypochondriack and Hysterick Passions.* London, 1711.

Marjara, Harinder Singh. *Contemplation of Created Things: Science and "Paradise Lost."* Buffalo: U of Toronto P, 1992.

Markley, Robert. *Fallen Languages: Crises of Representation in Newtonian England, 1660–1740.* Ithaca, N.Y.: Cornell UP, 1993.

————. "Objectivity as Ideology: Boyle, Newton, and the Languages of Science." *Genre* 16 (1983): 355–72.

————. "Representing Order: Natural Philosophy, Mathematics, and Theology in the Newtonian Revolution." In *Chaos and Order: Complex Dynamics in Literature and Science,* ed. N. Katherine Hayles, 125–48. Chicago: U of Chicago P, 1991.

————. "Robert Boyle on Language: Some Considerations Touching the Style of Holy Scriptures." *Studies in Eighteenth-Century Culture* 14 (1985): 159–71.

————. "Sentimentality as Performance: Shaftesbury, Sterne, and the Theatrics of Virtue." In *The New Eighteenth Century: Theory, Politics, English Literature,* ed. Felicity Nussbaum and Laura Brown. New York: Methuen, 1987.

Marwil, Jonathan. *The Trials of Counsel: Francis Bacon in 1621.* Detroit: Wayne State UP, 1976.

Marotti, Arthur F. "John Donne and the Rewards of Patronage." In *Patronage in the Renaissance,* ed. Guy Fitch Lytle and Stephen Orgel, 207–34. Princeton, N.J.: Princeton UP, 1981.

————. *John Donne, Coterie Poet.* Madison: U of Wisconsin P, 1986.

Martin, Julian. *Francis Bacon, the State and the Reform of Natural Philosophy.* Cambridge: Cambridge UP, 1992.

Mayr, Otto. *Authority, Liberty, and Automatic Machinery in Early Modern Europe.* Baltimore: Johns Hopkins UP, 1986.

Merchant, Carolyn. *The Death of Nature: Women, Ecology, and the Scientific Revolution.* 1980. Reprint. San Francisco: Harper & Row, 1989.

Merrens, Rebecca. "Exchanging Cultural Capital: Troping Women in Sidney and Bacon." *Genre* 25 (1992): 179–92.

Milton, John. *Complete Poems and Major Prose.* Ed. Merritt Hughes. New York: Odyssey Press, 1957.

————. *Paradise Lost.* Ed. Alastair Fowler. New York: Longman, 1968.

Montaigne, Michel. *The Essayes of Montaigne.* Trans. John Florio. 1604. New York: Random House, 1933.

Mueller, Janel. "Women among the Metaphysicals: A Case, Mostly, of Being Donne For." In *Critical Essays on John Donne*, ed. Arthur Mariotti, 37–48. New York: G. K. Hall, 1994.

Mullan, John. "Hypochondria and Hysteria: Sensibility and the Physicians." *Eighteenth Century* 25 (1984): 141–76.

————. *Sentiment and Sensibility: The Language of Feeling in the Eighteenth Century.* New York: Oxford UP, 1988.

Nicolson, Marjorie Hope. *The Breaking of the Circle: Studies in the Effect of the "New Science" upon Seventeenth-Century Poetry.* 2d ed. New York: Columbia UP, 1960.

————. *John Milton: A Reader's Guide to His Poetry.* New York: Farrar, Straus & Giroux, 1963.

————. *Science and Imagination.* 1936. Reprint. Ithaca, N.Y.: Great Seal Books, 1962.

Norbrook, David. "The Monarchy of Wit and the Republic of Letters: Donne's Politics." In *Soliciting Interpretation: Literary Theory and Seventeenth-Century English Poetry*, ed. Elizabeth Harvey and Katharine Eisaman Maus, 3–36. Chicago: U of Chicago P, 1990.

Oldenburg, Henry. *The Correspondence of Henry Oldenburg.* Ed. A. Rupert Hall. 11 vols. Madison: U of Wisconsin P, 1965–77.

Parisi, Hope. "Discourse and Danger: Women's Heroism in the Bible and Dalila's Self-Defense." In *Spokesperson Milton: Voices in Contemporary Criticism*, ed. Charles W. Durham and Kristin Pruitt McColgan, 260–74. Selingsgrove, Pa.: Susquehanna UP, 1994.

Parry, Graham. *The Golden Age Restor'd: The Culture of the Stuart Court, 1604–42.* Manchester: Manchester UP, 1981.

Patterson, Annabel. "All Donne." In *Soliciting Interpretation: Literary Theory and Seventeenth-Century English Poetry*, ed. Elizabeth Harvey and Katharine Eisaman Maus, 37–67. Chicago: U of Chicago P, 1990.

————. *Censorship and Interpretation: The Conditions of Writing and Reading in Early Modern Europe.* Madison: U of Wisconsin P, 1984.

————. "John Donne, Kingsman?" In *The Mental World of the Jacobean Court*, ed. Linda Levy Peck. New York: Cambridge UP, 1991.

Philips, Patricia. *The Scientific Lady: A Social History of Women's Scientific Interests, 1520–1918.* London: Weidenfeld & Nicolson, 1990.

Porter, Roy. *Mind-Forg'd Manacles: A History of Madness in England from the Restoration to the Regency.* London: Penguin Books, 1987.

Proctor, Robert. *Cancer Wars: How Politics Shapes What We Know and Don't Know about Cancer.* New York: Basic Books, 1995.

Puttenham, George. *The Arte of English Poesie.* Ed. Gladys Doidge Willcock and Alice Walker. Cambridge: Cambridge UP, 1936.

Quint, David. *Epic and Empire: Politics and Generic Form from Virgil to Milton.* Princeton, N.J.: Princeton UP, 1993.

Radzinowicz, Mary Ann. "Milton and the Tragic Women of Genesis." In *Essays on Milton and His World,* ed. P. G. Stanwood, 131–52. Binghamton, N.Y.: Medieval and Renaissance Texts and Studies, 1995.

———. "The Politics of *Paradise Lost.*" In *The Politics of Discourse,* ed. Kevin Sharpe and Steven N. Zwicker, 203–21. Berkeley and Los Angeles: U of California P, 1987.

Rajan, Balachandra. "Banyan Trees and Fig Leaves: Some Thoughts on Milton's India." In *Of Poetry and Politics: New Essays on Milton and His World,* ed. P. G. Stanwood, 213–28. Binghamton, N.Y.: Medieval and Renaissance Texts and Studies, 1995.

Rogers, John. *The Matter of Revolution: Science, Poetry, and Politics in the Age of Milton.* Ithaca, N.Y.: Cornell UP, 1996.

Rogers, Katherine M. "Finch's 'Candid Account' vs. Eighteenth-Century Theories of the Spleen." *Mosaic* 22 (1989): 17–27.

Rogers, Katherine M., and William McCarthy. *The Meridian Anthology of Early Women Writers: British Literary Women from Aphra Behn to Maria Edgeworth, 1660–1800.* New York: New American Library, 1987.

Ross, Alexander. *The New Planet No Planet, or The Earth No Wandering Star Except in the Wandring Heads of Galileans.* London, 1646.

Rouse, Joseph. *Knowledge and Power: Toward a Political Philosophy of Science.* Ithaca, N.Y.: Cornell UP, 1987.

———. "What Are Cultural Studies of Scientific Knowledge?" *Configurations* 1 (1992): 1–22.

Salvaggio, Ruth. *Enlightened Absence: Neoclassical Configurations of the Feminine.* Urbana: U of Illinois P, 1988.

Schiebinger, Londa. "The Anatomy of Difference: Race and Sex in Eighteenth-Century Science." *Eighteenth-Century Studies* 23 (1990): 387–405.

———. *The Mind Has No Sex? Women in the Origins of Modern Science.* Cambridge, Mass.: Harvard UP, 1989.

Schoenfeldt, Michael C. "'Among Unequals What Society?' Strategic Courtesy and Christian Humility in *Paradise Lost*." *Milton Studies* 28 (1992): 71–90.

———. "Gender and Conduct in *Paradise Lost*." In *Sexuality and Gender in Early Modern Europe: Institutions, Texts, Images*, ed. James Grantham Turner, 310–38. New York: Cambridge UP, 1993.

Schuler, Robert. *Francis Bacon and Scientific Poetry*. Philadelphia: Transactions of the American Philosophical Society, 1992.

Serres, Michel. *Hermes: Literature, Science, Philosophy*. Ed. Josue V. Harari and David F. Bell. Baltimore: Johns Hopkins UP, 1982.

Shami, Jeanne. "Kings and Desperate Men: John Donne Preaches at Court." *John Donne Journal* 6 (1987): 9–23.

Shapin, Steve. *The Social History of Truth: Civility and Science in Seventeenth-Century England*. Chicago: U of Chicago P, 1994.

Shapin, Steve, and Simon Schaffer. *Leviathan and the Air-Pump: Hobbes, Boyle, and the Experimental Life*. Princeton, N.J.: Princeton UP, 1985.

Shapiro, Barbara. *John Wilkins, 1614–1672: An Intellectual Biography*. Berkeley and Los Angeles: U of California P, 1969.

———. *Probability and Certainty in Seventeenth-Century England: A Study of the Relationships between Natural Philosophy, Science, History, Law, and Literature*. Princeton, N.J.: Princeton UP, 1983.

Shapiro, I. A. "The Mermaid Club." *Modern Language Review* 45 (1950): 6–17.

Sharrock, Robert. *The History of the Propagation and Improvement of Vegetables by the Concurrence of Art and Nature*. London, 1655.

Sidney, Sir Philip. *An Apologie for Poetrie*. Ed. Evelyn Shuckburgh. New York: Cambridge UP, 1951.

Slaughter, M. M. *Universal Languages and Scientific Taxonomy in the Seventeenth Century*. New York: Cambridge UP, 1982.

Smith, A. J. *Donne: Songs and Sonets* (London: Edward Arnold, 1964).

Smith, Nigel. *Literature and Revolution in England, 1640–1660*. New Haven, Conn.: Yale UP, 1994.

———, ed. *A Collection of Ranter Writings from the Seventeenth Century*. London: Junction Books, 1983.

Snider, Alvin. *Origin and Authority in Seventeenth-Century England: Bacon, Milton, and Butler*. Buffalo: U of Toronto P, 1994.

Solomon, Julie. *Objectivity in the Making: Francis Bacon and the Politics of Inquiry*. Baltimore: Johns Hopkins UP, 1998.

———. "To Know, to Fly, to Conjure: Situating Baconian Science at the Juncture of Early Modern Modes of Reading." *Renaissance Quarterly* 44 (1991): 513–58.

Sprat, Thomas. *The History of the Royal Society of London for the Improving of Natural Knowledge.* London, 1667.

Stepan, Nancy. "Race and Gender: The Role of Analogy in Science." *Isis* (1986): 261–77.

Stephenson, Raymond. "Richardson's 'Nerves': The Physiology of Sensibility in *Clarissa.*" *Journal of the History of Ideas* 44 (1988): 267–73.

Stevens, Paul. "*Paradise Lost* and the Colonial Imperative." *Milton Studies* 34 (1996): 3–21.

Stillman, Robert. *The New Philosophy and Universal Languages in Seventeenth-Century England: Bacon, Hobbes, and Wilkins.* Lewsiburgh, Pa.: Bucknell UP, 1995.

Strier, Richard. "Radical Donne: Satire III." *ELH* 60 (1993): 283–322.

Stukeley, William. *Of the Spleen.* London, 1723.

Svendsen, Kester. *Milton and Science.* Cambridge, Mass.: Harvard UP, 1956.

Sydenham, Thomas. *The Whole Works of That Excellent Practial Physician, Dr. Thomas Sydenham.* Trans. John Pechy. London, 1696.

Tayler, Edward. *Donne's Idea of a Woman: The Structure and Meaning of the "Anniversaries."* New York: Columbia UP, 1991.

Toulmin, Stephen. "The Construal of Reality: Criticism in Modern and Postmodern Science." *Critical Inquiry* 9 (1982): 93–111.

Trotter, David. *The Poetry of Abraham Cowley.* New York: Macmillan, 1979.

U.S. Senate Committee on Labor and Human Resources. *Oversight of the Healthy Start Demonstration Project: Hearing before the Committee on Labor and Human Resources.* 104th Cong., 2d sess., 16 May 1996.

Vickers, Brian. "The Royal Society and English Prose Style: A Reassessment." In *Rhetoric and the Pursuit of Truth: Language and Change in the Seventeenth and Eighteenth Centuries,* ed. Brian Vickers and Nancy Streuver. Los Angeles: Clark Library, 1985.

Webster, Charles. *The Great Instauration: Science, Medicine, and Reform, 1626–1660.* New York: Holmes & Meier, 1976.

Westfall, Richard. *Science and Religion in Seventeenth-Century England.* New Haven, Conn.: Yale UP, 1958.

Westman, Robert S. "The Astronomer's Role in the Sixteenth Century: A Preliminary Study." *History of Science* 18 (1980): 105–46.

Whitney, Charles. *Francis Bacon and Modernity.* New Haven, Conn.: Yale UP, 1986.

Wilding, Michael. *Dragon's Teeth: Literature in the English Revolution.* Oxford: Clarendon Press, 1987.

———. "'Thir Sex Not Equal Seem'd': Equality in *Paradise Lost.*" In *Of Poetry and Politics: New Essays on Milton and His World,* ed. P. G. Stanwood, 172–85. Binghamton, N.Y.: Medieval and Renaissance Texts and Studies, 1995.

Wilkins, John. *A Discourse Concerning the Beauty of Providence.* London, 1649.

———. *The Discovery of a World in the Moone, or A Discourse Tending to Prove That 'Tis Probable There May Be Another Habitable World in That Planet.* London, 1638. Facs. ed. with introduction by Barbara Shapiro. Delmar, N.Y.: Scholars' Facsimile Reprints, 1973.

———. *Of the Principles and Duties of Natural Religion.* London, 1675.

Willis, Thomas. *The London Practice of Physick, or The Whole Practical Part of Physick Contained in the Works of Dr. Willis.* 1685. 2nd ed. London, 1689.

Wittreich, Joseph. "'Inspired with Contradiction': Mapping Gender Discourses in *Paradise Lost.*" In *Literary Milton: Text, Pretext, Context,* ed. Diana T. Benet and Michael Liebs, 133–61. Pittsburgh: Duquesne UP, 1994.

World Health Organization. *The Prevention of Cancer.* Geneva: WHO, 1964.

Yates, Frances A. *Astraea: The Imperial Theme in the Sixteenth-Century.* Boston: Routledge & Kegan Paul, 1975.

INDEX

Evelyn, John, *Sylva*, 124
Excellency of Theology, 13, 106, 126
Experiment, 18–19, 39–40, 51, 54, 83,
    89–90, 96–97, 143–44, 149, 164

Fallon, Stephen, 127
Finch, Anne, Countess of Winchilsea,
    5, 13, 18–21, 141–49, 152, 154–72;
    class in, 141, 147, 148, 157, 158, 159,
    165, 166–67, 170, 176; contingency
    in, 18– 19, 20, 142, 143–44,
    160–61, 171; Cowley, critique of,
    142, 143–46, 158–59, 161– 63;
    handmaid, trope of, 170, 176; on
    monarchy, 161, 163–67; and the
    Royal Society, 142, 144, 156,
    163–64; "the spleen," ideological
    critique of, 141–45, 148–49, 152,
    154–58, 161, 162–67, Sydenham,
    critique of, 142, 148, 154–58,
    161–64, 167; and voluntarism,
    144, 164; women and nature in,
    162–64; women's health care in,
    141, 142, 144, 148–49, 152, 154–58,
    161, 162–67; on women's writing,
    143, 146–47, 158–59, 164–67
    POEMS: "Ardelia to Melancholy,"
    142; "Circuit of Appollo, The,"
    146; "Introduction, The," 146,
    159; "Spleen, The," 141–47,
    148–49, 154–66
Frank, Robert, 191–92n.33
Freud, Sigmund, 166

Galen, 162
Galileo, *Sidereus Nuncius*, 8–9, 34–38

Gilbert, Sandra, 19
Gilbert, William, 13; *De Magnete*, 37, 52,
    83–85
Gildon, Charles, 187n.2
Golden Age, 49, 55, 79–80, 146
Good Old Cause, 155
Gould, Stephen J., 175n.25
Green, Robert, *Friar Bacon and Friar
    Bungay*, 26
Gubar, Susan, 19
Guerrini, Anita, 192n.33
Guibbory, Achsah, 63–64
Guillory, John, 182n.4, 186n.46

Hall, Joseph, 69–70
Handmaid, trope of, 14, 177; in Bacon,
    10–11, 13, 42–43; in Boyle, 13,
    126–27; and Finch, 170, 177
Haraway, Donna, 3, 168–70, 173n.1
Harland, Paul, 15, 31
Harrington, Lucy, Countess of
    Bedford, 68
Harrington, William, 24
Hartlib, Samuel, 17, 103–104, 122–24,
    184n.32
Harvey, William, 161, 164
Haydn, Hiram, 55
Henry, Prince of Wales, 54–68, 97,
    180n.8
Higginson, John, 6
Hill, Christopher, 9, 127, 129, 169,
    174nn.10,11, 182n.4
Hinnant, Charles, 141–42
Hobbes, Thomas, 18, 106, 112, 119
Hoby, Edward, 34
Hooke, Robert, 192n.33